Acclaim for The Fertility Guide:

Information, communication and guidance. These were the three most important factors to us as we began our treatment. Our physician not only answered questions but offered information on issues ranging from treatment options for becoming pregnant to what our treatment options would cost.

I hope this book will become one every OB/Gyn gives to a patient he/she is referring to a fertility specialist, for I found it to be an extremely comprehensive, informative and understandable guide to the treatment process.

-Annette Discerni Wilson

What makes it stand out from other infertility books is its coverage of the emotional as well as medical aspects of infertility. . . describes in clear, concise terms how it feels to go through the infertility evaluation and treatment...the reader is assured that the authors understand all the facets of the infertility experience...it allows the patient to be an active and informed participant in their treatment process ..increases their feelings of control over the treatment process... I will routinely recommend it to the couples I work with.

-Susan C. Klock, Ph.D.
Assistant Professor of Obstetrics,
Gynecology and Psychiatry
Northwestern University
Medical School

*This book is an excellent resource for couples facing infertility issues. Dr. Jarrett is an extremely competent and caring Reproductive Endocrinologist who clearly explains the most current medical procedures available. Dr. Rausch provides warmth and understanding when helping patients deal with accompanying emotions. I highly recommend **The Fertility Guide.***

-Ann

The joint efforts of Dr. Rausch, who addresses the emotional side of infertility coupled with Dr. Jarrett's chapters on the medical issues and treatments involved make this book a valuable resource for couples. It is written in easy to understand language and at the same time answers all your questions about tests, results and what they mean to you. I recommend this book to our readers.

-Barbara Nesbitt
Editor, OBGYN.net

THE FERTILITY GUIDE:

A COUPLES HANDBOOK FOR WHEN YOU WANT TO HAVE A BABY (MORE THAN ANYTHING ELSE)

John C. Jarrett II, M.D.
Deidra T. Rausch, Ph.D.

Health Press
Santa Fe, NM
www.healthpress.com

Published by Health Press
P.O. Box 1388
Santa Fe, NM 87504
www.healthpress.com

ISBN 09-929173-2-95

Library of Congress Cataloging-in-Publication Data

Jarrett, John C., 1950-
　　The fertility guide: a couples handbook for when you want to have a baby (more than anything else) / John C. Jarrett II, Deidra T. Rausch.
　　　　　p.　cm.
　　ISBN 0-929173-29-5 (trade paper)
　　1. Infertility--Popular works.　I. Rausch, Deidra T., 1961-
II. Title.
RC889.J37 1998　　　　　　　　　　　97-35087
616.6'92--DC21　　　　　　　　　　　CIP

Printed in the United States of America

10 9 8 7 6 5 4 3 2

DEDICATION

To my father, for being such a great role model
To my mother, for never-ending love and support
To my wife, for her unwavering belief and efforts,
and to my kids, for their understanding

JCJ

ACKNOWLEDGMENTS

I feel privileged to have accompanied so many couples as they navigate the infertility journey. Through our experiences over the past eleven years I have been able to observe different aspects of the journey and am excited about the opportunity to share some helpful hints for survival. I have been surrounded by supportive people throughout my life journey, and offer special thanks to Dave, Taylor, Meredith, Jake and my parents Tom and Jeanine for their patience and support.

DR

UNCHARTED TERRITORY

How can I say good-bye,
When we've not yet said hello?

My "Imagined Child" — will you ever come to be?

From early years the future was guaranteed--now
I wonder, "Will this dream be realized?"

Carefree and assured, we started our lives together;
Tentative and unsure, will we forever fear the future?

The pathway to you is uncertain,
The questions unanswerable.

As the journey continues, filled with evaluation of
uncharted territory, my vision of you remains constant.

My peace is found in knowing that while I may not
hold you in my arms, I will always hold you in my heart.

D. Rausch

TABLE OF CONTENTS

INTRODUCTION

Infertility is a term that strikes fear in the hearts of every couple who worries it may, or learns that it does, apply to them. Ten to fifteen percent of all couples, or as many as 2.5 million American couples, hear this diagnosis and must begin the frustrating and sometimes arduous journey of receiving medical help and undergoing treatment to achieve what should be one of life's most basic and simple accomplishments—having a baby.

But if you are one of these couples, there is good news—and the news is getting better all the time. In the last ten years our understanding of human conception, and our ability to assist couples who have difficulty conceiving, has grown exponentially. Not only can the vast majority of couples with infertility now conceive, but they can do so with less testing and fewer invasive procedures than previously. *The treatment of infertility can be less expensive, take less time, and be tremendously more successful than ever before.*

This book fills an important void. It is written for you, the average couple who want to understand your problem. It provides clear and simple information. It outlines what steps are reasonable, what tests make sense, and what treatments are worthwhile. It also discusses ways you can cope with emotional aspects of the infertility journey.

The Fertility Guide will:

- Define fertility problems in clear and simple terms that every couple can understand.

- Explain the treatment options available for each particular problem.

- Improve your ability to participate in your own care because you will understand both the problem(s) and the available treatment options.

- Explain why the treatment of infertility has changed dramatically in the last few years.

- Detail why certain costly and invasive procedures, *e.g.*, diagnostic laparoscopy, should no longer be a routine part of fertility evaluation.

- Suggest ways to adjust to the emotional aspects of infertility.

The Fertility Guide has a bias. We believe that the evaluation and treatment of impaired fertility *does not* need to:

- Take forever

- Be nearly as invasive as it has been in the past

- Be financially devastating

- Ruin marriages

- Ruin one's self-esteem

For those couples who have not yet begun to undergo an infertility evaluation, this book begins with a discussion of the emotional states you may experience in navigating the process. It also provides guidelines to follow as you undergo your evaluation. You can become your own advocates and can participate with your physician in a truly informed fashion as to the steps you are willing to pursue.

For couples who have already undergone much of this evaluation, this book is not intended to make you second-guess the steps that have already been taken, nor to feel poorly about the choices you have made in the past. (Never second-guess the decisions and choices you make, but do make every effort to be sure that you make the best ones you can.) It is intended to make options clearly understood and to provide a framework for continued pursuit of fertility.

It is our belief that infertility teams providing treatment must attend to both the medical and emotional aspects of this life experience. For this reason, *The Fertility Guide* is separated into three sections. In the first short section Dr. Rausch will take you through the emotional aspects of infertility with helpful advice for navigating the emotional journey. Dealing with the emotional aspects of infertility is every bit as important as correcting the physical problem. While both aspects must be addressed by your infertility treatment team for a successful outcome, remember your emotions will act as a filter through which you will experience the physical aspects, and therefore must be openly addressed.

In the second section Dr. Jarrett deals with the "nuts and bolts" of the physical aspects of infertility—the various causes of difficulty conceiving and the treatment alternatives.

Finally, many couples feel it is helpful to keep track of their evaluation and treatment as they attempt to conceive. Easy to use, organized flow sheets are provided in the third section at the end of this book, which will help you record your results and track your evaluation. Recording this information will be helpful to you and your physicians.

Read this book. Use it.

You will develop a better understanding of your problem(s), a better awareness of the evaluation options available, and a better ability to participate in informed decisions as to which treatments to pursue. It will make your efforts more tolerable, less expensive, less time consuming, and more successful. *You need to be involved in charting your course as you pursue fertility.* This book will help you do so.

PART I:
UNDERSTANDING THE EMOTIONAL
ASPECTS OF INFERTILITY

Deidra T. Rausch, Ph.D.

Dr. Jarrett will take you through the physical/medical side of the infertility treatment in Part II of *The Fertility Guide*. Now, however, it's important that you clearly understand our belief that infertility is both a medical and emotional experience. Our team at Midwest Reproductive Medicine includes health care professionals who focus on the medical treatment of infertility, as well as provide counseling services to address the emotional aspects of this life experience. We strongly feel programs that exclude a focus on the psychosocial components of infertility are not providing you with comprehensive care.

For more than ten years I have worked with couples facing the challenge of infertility. My initial role as a nurse required significant focus on the procedural aspects of infertility. It was important to be sure patients were called, ultrasounds performed, and surgeries scheduled. Yet during an ultrasound exam, taking patients back to consult rooms to wait for the physician, or calling patients with pregnancy test results, it was evident to me that the emotional aspects of infertility were of equal significance. It became quite apparent that the ability to physically tolerate procedures was often easier than tolerating the emotions that accompanied the treatment. Patients would say, "At least when I'm taking fertility meds and doing ultrasounds I'm doing something. That two-week wait to find out leaves me out of control and is unbearable!"

Over the last five years I have served as the counselor on our infertility team. I am fortunate to have time to just sit with clients to listen to what they say the emotional experience of infertility is like for them. The overwhelming emotion they say is created by infertility is "loss."

Potential losses associated with infertility include: 1) the loss of feeling normal, 2) the loss of self-esteem, 3) the loss of friendships, 4) the loss of relationships with family members, 5) the loss of control over life events, and 6) the loss of privacy. After all, if given a choice, who would want a medical team to invade the privacy of their bedroom?

Certainly it is great that technology is available to help couples that previously did not have hope to parent genetically, yet the need to utilize procedures often stirs feelings of grief. Often patients will express frustration with others who suggest that they should be excited or happy to be doing infertility treatments. Though you might be grateful the treatments exist, it's perceived as a loss to have to welcome an infertility team into your baby-making world.

An awareness of all the losses that you and your partner are experiencing is the first step to emotionally winning this battle. Our commitment as an infertility team is to the belief that infertility is a couple's issue, not just the issue of the partner bearing the medical diagnosis. Evidence has shown that couples who are committed to working together and supporting each other through this process fare best.

Throughout the following section the emotional aspects of infertility will be explored with helpful advice in navigating the emotional journey as a couple. In addition to evaluating the emotional response to infertility, I will also discuss the psychosocial aspects that accompany the transition, as well as alternatives to parenting such as donor gametes, adoption, child-free living, and single-child parenting. Finally an evaluation of pregnancy after infertility will be addressed with attention to the emotions involved in this move from the infertile to fertile world.

While the second section of *The Fertility Guide* will help you understand how to be an active, informed participant in your "medical" evaluation and treatment, this section will help you do the same for the emotional hurdles you may encounter, enabling you to understand them, deal with them, and be stronger because of your efforts.

CHAPTER ONE
NAVIGATING THE EMOTIONAL JOURNEY

For many couples the experience of infertility is the first life crisis they must confront together. Often we have expectations that pregnancy can be controlled. Early in the marriage or relationship birth control is available to prevent pregnancy, so it is assumed that when the time is right pregnancy will happen. The realization that there might be a fertility problem comes as a shock.

Rarely are we educated that one out of ten couples have difficulties becoming pregnant. And typically you assume that you will not be that one unlucky couple. Couples who have been surrounded by fertile friends and families may have increased levels of shock as compared to those who have shared infertility experiences with others. Regardless, the diagnosis of infertility is often a cruel awakening.

It is important at this point in the journey for you to allow each other to feel the grief and frustration that naturally accompanies the realization that parenting may be more challenging than you expected. The grief of "not getting pregnant the old-fashioned way" is normal and needs to be discussed. Taking time to attend to the shock and disappointment that each of you may be feeling is vital to future coping abilities throughout infertility treatment.

DENIAL

Denial is often considered a negative coping mechanism. In many cases denial can actually assist you in pursuing treatment with optimism. Often couples do appear to be starting "down the creek without a paddle," due to lack of communication about the fertility issues.

For many couples, the experience of infertility is the first time in their lifes when they are unable to control the outcome. Often, the "if I work hard, I'll get it" philosophy serves as a motivation for pursuit of solutions. This commitment feels good if each partner shares the same beliefs with respect to potential treatments.

Denial can be a negative experience if each partner is in a different place with respect to optimism for the future. It is not uncommon for one partner to believe pregnancy is going to happen, while the other is filled with the belief that treatment will prove futile.

One way to help address this discrepancy is to develop a relationship with a physician who can give you honest information with regard to procedures and the realistic opportunity for success. When the pursuit of treatment is discouraged, continued use of denial can cause couples to "doctor shop" in an effort to find someone who will fix their infertility.

Couples who experience continued inability to accept the infertility diagnosis, or are feeling different with respect to optimism for pregnancy, often find counseling beneficial. Counselors can serve as translators of medical information and provide a neutral sounding board for couples to discuss differences.

ANGER

Anger is a very normal response to infertility. This can be directed toward a variety of individuals, including your partner, self, friends, family, medical providers and even spiritually. It is not uncommon for feelings of anger to occur when pregnancies are announced by friends and families, or when past experiences have caused your partner's infertility. Also, when previous health care providers have ignored concerns about fertility or have been slow to refer you to a specialist, anger with respect to their role in your infertility is common. Finally, those strongly religious individuals who have lived with the belief "if I'm a good person, bad things won't happen" can be angry about the lack of ability to control parenting.

Culturally, it is more common for men to express their anger and for women to suppress it. It is important each of you talk about your feelings and find ways to express your anger directly. Often exercise can help release the tension caused by anger. Many times anger does a great job of covering up other emotions that are difficult to express. Spending time clarifying your emotions, either alone or with a therapist, can help to diffuse the intensity of anger.

WHY ME?

Questioning why infertility happens is normal. We live in a country that upholds the "cause and effect principle," therefore, searching for answers comes naturally. So the ability to accept randomness is foreign and often uncomfortable.

Infertility often poses the first threat to our belief that we can control life events. This desire for control is not uncommon. Typically our past efforts have always led us to believe we do have control over life events. Infertility experiences bring our control into question, and can lead to increased anxiety about other areas of life. I call this the *mushroom effect*.

In order to prevent the mushroom effect from occurring it is beneficial to acknowledge areas of your life that you do control and accept those that you can't. For some individuals turning toward spirituality can provide comfort and support in the process of letting go of the need to control. Often one of the benefits of infertility is the opportunity to develop a greater appreciation for life. The knowledge that sometimes bad things can happen often inspires an increased enjoyment in good things when they occur.

BLAME AND GUILT

Many times the quest for an explanation for the infertility can lead to self-blame. Individuals who have experienced a sexually transmitted disease, abortion, sterilization, or thoughts of never wanting children are at increased risk for feelings of blame or guilt. Taking on feelings of blame and guilt can lead to decreased self-esteem. Therefore, it is important to challenge negative thoughts.

Remember that it's always easy to come up with a better answer after we see the result of our previous decisions. Yet, second-guessing does more harm than good.

For some couples unspoken feelings of blame and guilt can lead to marital sabotage. Sometimes one partner makes a decision that the other deserves a better life and an opportunity to parent. In an effort to make this happen they will either ask for a divorce, or make life so difficult that the other partner is forced to leave. Remember that you are together because you love each other and wanted to share your lives, not for each other's reproductive capacity.

Unresolved blame and guilt can cause you to feel stuck. This can lead to an unending pursuit of treatment for self-punishment, or refusal to try treatments because of a belief that you don't deserve to be a parent. When feelings of blame and guilt are deeply ingrained, it is beneficial to explore counseling in an effort to better understand the impact these emotions can have on you and your relationship.

ISOLATION

Infertility is a personal experience. Often couples are uncomfortable discussing their fertility with others. Issues of embarrassment talking about sexuality and reproduction, and feelings of inadequacy or shame can lead to cutting off potential support of others.

Many times being around others who have children can be a source of pain. The reminder that "they have what I want" often leads to sadness and jealousy, and, ultimately, a distancing in the relationship. Unfortunately, elimination of social connections can lead to increased isolation and lack of support.

Be aware of your reasons for distancing yourself from friends, family and colleagues. There certainly are people who "just don't understand" and can say hurtful things. With some education and direct communication you will find that friends and family do want to help, but just don't know how. Remember that direct communication of your needs benefits both you and those who wish to help.

I certainly don't advocate discussion of your situation with everyone. It is a good idea to consider which individuals are support systems, and which are systems that you are supporting. Typically if someone is willing to just listen and respond to your needs, they are supportive. On the other hand, if you find yourself "acting fine" or saying "I'm doing great" when in fact you're not, that is someone you are supporting.

Support groups can be very helpful in decreasing the feeling "that we're the only ones who can't get pregnant." Often you may feel that no one else has ever been infertile. Support groups can be helpful in normalizing the prevalence of infertility and your emotional responses to this experience.

MAINTAINING RELATIONSHIP COHESION

The experience of infertility differs from one individual to the next. Often when partners feel differently about the ability to achieve fertility, feelings of isolation increase. It is important to consider these differences in order to understand each other better.

Men frequently have a double agenda when it comes to infertility. They are often focused on achieving a pregnancy as well as taking care of their partner. Historically, men have been trained to "kill the bear and take care of the woman." This ideal automatically creates the tendency for men to "try to fix it." Additionally, society often teaches men they should be strong and not show emotions, leaving them with anger as the only emotion they feel acceptable to express.

For most women society has granted permission to express a variety of emotions. Crying and talking about the pain of not being able to achieve pregnancy is acceptable. Women are able to focus solely on the pursuit of the child and don't have the dual responsibility of worrying about themselves.

Many times women just want to be able to talk about the infertility and don't expect answers or cures. But for men, processing feelings and thoughts is often an internal process. When they talk, they want feedback or action.

These differences are important to acknowledge. You don't want to fall into a pattern of assuming you know what your partner needs or wants, rather than asking.

It often helps to remember the phrase "to understand does not mean to agree." If you can work toward not expecting your partner to feel the way you do, but rather expect they can accept the way you feel as valid, your relationship will be on solid ground. Increased conversations about the feelings that result from being at different places with respect to emotions and decision making is vital to maintaining relationship cohesion.

INTIMACY

Infertility poses a great threat to the intimacy experienced by couples. So often making love is equated to making babies. As infertility persists, the feeling of failure can invade your sexual relationship and cause intercourse to be a painful reminder of what is not happening.

Additionally, some procedures cause increased ovarian size, which makes intercourse uncomfortable and in some cases prohibited. Remember, there is more to intimacy than intercourse. It's not uncommon for couples to forget to express their affection or assume their partner "knows I love him/her." During infertility treatments, it is essential for you to increase your affection and verbal commitment to each other.

Often the best gift you can give your relationship is time out from treatment. Breaks from a treatment regimen give you the opportunity to refuel your "emotional bank account" and take time for each other. Remember, you came together for what you saw in each other, not just for children you might have together.

GRIEF

Often society does not acknowledge grief over the inability to have children, although this grief is valid. Each cycle without pregnancy is often experienced as the death of hopes and dreams. Just as with other losses this causes grief—but often it is more difficult to resolve. The grief of infertility is "ambiguous." There is no "body" and often there is not an arena for expression of this grief with others.

Many times acknowledging the painful feelings that are associated with negative pregnancy tests or periods that start is the first step to grief resolution. It may also be helpful to write down what a positive pregnancy test would have meant and what this child would have been like. Though these exercises sound painful, they help make your loss concrete, which increases your permission to yourself to grieve.

Discounting the significance of a treatment cycle does not cause the pain to be any less if it is unsuccessful. This practice simply makes it more difficult to allow yourself to feel the true pain of disappointment and lost hope for the attempt. In addition, the accumulation of unresolved grief makes it more and more difficult to continue on after a time.

You will each experience the grief of infertility differently. Be honest with yourself and your partner and decide what you need to do to heal from the disappointments of infertility. Many patients find it is helpful to talk to counselors who have previously worked with infertile couples. The ability to discuss the feelings of loss associated with reproductive disappointments can be very healing.

DEPRESSION

Depression is a natural emotion to experience when grieving. Many couples fear they will never be happy again. Also, if this is the first loss that has been experienced, the feeling of depression can be very scary. Oftentimes the ability to talk about disappointments and feelings of loss help alleviate the depression.

Couples frequently expect themselves to "snap back to normal" more quickly than is realistic. It is unrealistic to assume you will feel happy the day after a negative pregnancy test or miscarriage. By reminding yourself this cycle was filled with hopes and dreams, you can validate the presence of depression.

If the depression persists for a long period of time, leading to physical illness or feelings of hopelessness, it is important for you to talk with a counselor. Occasionally, it might be suggested you take a break from treatments and consider medications to assist in decreasing the depression.

RESOLUTION

Resolution occurs at different points for different couples. Many times the availability of treatments makes it difficult to stop before you've done everything you can do. It is important for you to always have a positive reason for pursuing treatment in addition to pregnancy. Some couples discover early in the fertility pursuit that it is time to stop, while others find it important to pursue all possible technologies. There is no right or wrong time to stop. Each of you must talk about your hopes and expectations and ultimately reach a decision together.

Once a decision to stop occurs, work through the grief that is experienced. After processing the grief of infertility, resolution does occur. You may feel that you will never be the same again. Many times it is easier to focus on the negative effects of infertility and lose sight of the positive aspects that have been learned. Broadening your definition of success is significant in your ability to embrace the positive aspects of the infertility experience.

For many couples infertility causes positive change in the relationship. Often you are forced to learn new communication skills in order to survive the fertility pursuit. Infertility is typically the first life crisis a couple has endured together, so you learn more about ways to work as a team when facing difficulties. This skill will serve you in the years to come.

Not only do you learn new coping skills as a couple, but individual styles of coping are also gained with infertility. We don't come equipped with instructions for "Grief 101." Often we learn how to deal with disappointments by enduring them. The infertility experience certainly helps add new tools to your "grief resolution toolbox."

Finally, the pursuit of fertility does increase our appreciation for aspects of life that previously were outside of our awareness. Couples who have experienced infertility rarely take life for granted. Parenting experiences often hold special joys that otherwise might have been overlooked. Infertility definitely causes individuals to appreciate the moment because of an increased awareness that the future cannot always be controlled.

Chapter Two
Evaluating the Alternatives

Once you make a decision to stop pursuing medical treatment and resolve the grief of infertility, it is important to evaluate alternatives to genetic parenting. This chapter will explore the psychosocial aspects of adoption, donor gametes, child-free living, and single-child parenting.

Adoption

Couples who reassess their goals with respect to parenting and find they desire "a" child, not necessarily "our" child, often grieve the genetic dream child and pregnancy experience. Then they explore adoption. Adoption does provide more of a guarantee that parenting will occur than does treatment, but the emotional journey also has some ups and downs. The move from the familiar world of infertility treatments to the unknown arena of adoption can be overwhelming. It is not uncommon for family and friends to encourage the infertile couple to adopt. Stories of pregnancy after adoption abound and often are shared with the infertile. Certainly this can occur, but only does so in about 2% of the cases. A prevalent social assumption is that if a couple has pursued treatment unsuccessfully, then they will adopt.

The increased presence of private attorneys and agencies has decreased the waiting time for adoption, but costs can sometimes become prohibitive for many couples. On the average, the cost of adoption ranges from $10,000 to $25,000 depending on the age and ethnicity of the child. Often couples must regroup financially after exploring fertility treatments before they can realistically consider adoption.

Home studies can seem intimidating as couples wonder about their "marketability" to birth mothers and adoption facilitators. The idea of being *approved* to parent often brings feelings of resentment and frustration. The ability to write "Dear Birth Mother" letters stating all the positive qualities possessed by the couple can be difficult if self-esteem is low following the pursuit of fertility.

Adoptions that fall through after couples have been matched with birth parents sometimes feel like *déjà vu* with respect to previous miscarriages and unsuccessful cycles. Most adoption facilitators do a good job of preparing couples for possible disappointment, and remind them that with perseverance success is possible.

For those of you who have spent time together evaluating your motivations and desires for parenting and utilize reputable agencies, adoption can be a very positive experience. Often the excitement of knowing "we will be parents" is a refreshing change from the uncertainties of the treatment experience.

Presently the current depiction of adoption by the media creates a very scary picture. Many times couples discount the adoption alternative for fear a child will be taken away from them in the years ahead, or the child will ultimately seek out his or her birth parents. In order to make an informed decision, we suggest that even couples who feel adoption is not for them contact adoption attorneys and agencies so their decision is made in an informed manner, just as the fertility treatment decisions were made.

DONOR GAMETES

Sometimes the alternative of donor sperm or donor eggs will be suggested by the physician. You need to recognize the use of donor gametes as an *alternative form* of parenting. Difficulties can arise if you perceive the use of donor as a *treatment* for infertility. As with the other alternatives, grieving is important for your transition to and acceptance of donor sperm or eggs.

You will need to reevaluate your goals, and know that genetic parenting will not occur. Often a desire to know half of the genetics and to have a pregnancy experience makes the use of donor more optimal than adoption. You and your partner must evaluate the inequity of the genetic contribution. Those who experience feelings of "if not mine, then neither of ours" would do best to pursue adoption or child-free living.

Sperm banks provide couples with a variety of choices with respect to potential donors, yet the same is not so with respect to egg donors. Because of this lack of selection, some couples decide to use known donors. There are positives and negatives associated with this decision. It is often comforting to know the personality, medical, and psychological history of the donor, but uncertainty about potential custody issues exist. The opportunity for privacy is also compromised when a choice is made to use a known donor.

Consideration of disclosure versus nondisclosure is important prior to pursuing a donor. You and your partner need to make preliminary decisions about whether or not the potential child will know about the use of a donor. Discussion of this issue is best facilitated by your evaluations of comfort with secrets and consideration of whether or not it is a child's right to know their genetic origin.

Couples who decide not to tell the child are advised to tell no one in order to prevent concern over accidental disclosure in the future. Those couples who decide to tell the child are encouraged to have this discussion prior to the child's identity formation in adolescence.

CHILD-FREE LIVING

When the goal continues to remain "our" child, and a couple makes the decision to stop treatment, the alternative which presents is child-free living. The decision to live without children in the home is different from being childless. A couple must grieve their infertility and then consciously decide their lives will not have a parenting focus.

This alternative is often challenged by the societal emphasis to parent. You can be pressured to conform and be labeled as "selfish" if you choose to live without children. Additionally, you can feel internal pressure to do "Nobel prize" level activities in order to balance the inability to have genetic children.

Because you and your partner can differ in your commitment to child-free living it is imperative that honest communication of feelings occur. Research has demonstrated men typically are more comfortable than women with the option of child-free living. For those of you who do choose to pursue a child-free life style, fulfillment will come from personal and career accomplishments.

SINGLE-CHILD PARENTING

Couples experiencing secondary infertility may decide to stop treatment and focus on single-child parenting. Many times the pressure to have a second child in order to provide a sibling is tremendous. Often these couples are told countless times, "You should be grateful, at least you have one." Though this may be true, the motivation to pursue additional pregnancies is more concrete—a desire to do it again prevails.

You and your partner must evaluate the toll of treatment on your relationship with your existing child and the physical, financial and emotional costs of continued treatment. Increased understanding of the dynamics of raising an "only child" is important so that you don't buy into the typical stereotype of the spoiled, only child. Again, seeking the counsel of a therapist can be very valuable in making this decision.

Single-child parenting allows you to invest wholeheartedly in your child's life. Often extra effort to provide opportunities for interaction with other children occurs. Additionally, single-child parenting may create greater financial freedom. Though children often persist in their request for a sibling, ultimately the ability of their parents to grieve the inability to have a second child through to resolution will provide them with the opportunity to enjoy their family of three.

CHAPTER THREE
PREGNANCY AFTER INFERTILITY

After experiencing infertility it can be difficult to believe a positive pregnancy test can really be true. Initially, many couples are thrilled to hear they have finally succeeded, but quickly you may be filled with fears about the preciousness of the pregnancy. It is difficult to transition from the experience of treatments that may not have worked and the conditioned learning to "expect nothing," to acceptance that the pregnancy is real.

If you have had previous pregnancy losses, you may be unable to accept the possibility that this time may be different. Increased discussions about the fear of being optimistic and believing parenting can occur is beneficial for you and your partner. Sometimes the belief "if we think it will happen then it won't," or, conversely, "if we think it won't happen then it will" is present. This can interfere with your ability to enjoy the pregnancy experience.

Many times the fear of miscarriage can influence your decision to reveal your pregnancy to others. You and your partner may experience a wide variety of emotions ranging from frustration that your family isn't worried to disappointment in their cautious lack of excitement. Direct communication of needs and expectations to your support persons is necessary so they know what to say and do.

It is not unusual to postpone shopping for maternity clothes or baby items until well into the second, or even third, trimester. Thoughts may persist that "if we don't get excited and miscarriage happens, it won't hurt as much." Ultimately this can deprive both of you the joy of the early months of pregnancy and adjustment to parenting.

If you can allow yourselves to enjoy each day of the pregnancy experience, you will create positive memories that will serve you regardless of the pregnancy outcome. Many times the use of positive statements helps to decrease the anxiety you may be feeling . A conscious effort to challenge thoughts of "what if a miscarriage occurs" with statements of "everything is going as it should" can help to restructure any negative thinking.

You may find that relationships established with other infertile couples are threatened with the news of pregnancy. It is important for couples to have discussions about the issues of pregnancy early in your friendship, addressing the need for honesty about conflicting feelings of joy and jealousy which may occur with pregnancy. The transition from the infertile to the fertile world can be scary. You should try to maintain as many support systems as possible.

Leaving the comfort and familiarity of the infertility practice for the obstetrician's office can also be stressful. Relationships with the infertility team are often strong and the thought of not seeing "your team" on a regular basis can cause sadness. You may feel uneasy about the "laid back" nature of the obstetrical practice. You and your partner should schedule a consultation early on with the obstetrician to discuss anxieties and the "precious nature" of the pregnancy. You may ask for increased office visits during the early months of pregnancy to discuss anxiety and expectations of the prenatal experience. In time, as you become familiar with the various staff members your comfort should increase.

Frequent discussions with your partner about the excitement and anxiety of the pregnancy helps to normalize each other's feelings. You might consider keeping a journal of the pregnancy experience to document the memories for yourselves and the future child. Allow yourself to accept invitations for baby showers and other celebrations. The benefits of allowing yourselves to believe parenting will happen is greater than any risk of "jinxing" the pregnancy.

Sometimes the fact you wanted to get pregnant so desperately will create a resistance to complain about the negative effects of pregnancy, such as morning sickness, weight gain, and stretch marks. The same hesitancy may exist when the baby is born and you feel you can't express your frustration at lack of sleep and uncertainty with parenting skills. Remember that you are human, and it is all right if you don't feel happy about every single aspect of pregnancy and parenting. Don't set unrealistic goals.

Ultimately, the previous infertility experience can create an increased appreciation for parenting due to the realization that pregnancy is not a given. Evaluation of your motivations to parent throughout the course of the infertility experience provides you and your partner with a clear understanding of why you both want children and increases your abilities to enjoy parenting more fully.

PART II:
UNDERSTANDING THE MEDICAL ASPECTS OF INFERTILITY

THE PHYSICAL "NUTS AND BOLTS"

CHAPTER FOUR
NATURE'S WAY

Human conception is an elegantly simple and marvelously complex series of events. Before we can begin to discuss the reasons certain couples have difficulty conceiving, it is important to have a full understanding of the way things are supposed to work. A good working knowledge of normal events will make the steps that can be taken to evaluate a couple's fertility make more sense. Understanding "nature's way" will also provide a framework for understanding the rationale behind some of the therapeutic measures that will be discussed later.

THE MALE AND THE SPERM

Sperm are constantly being produced in the testicles of the adult male. This process begins at puberty and continues throughout the remainder of the man's life. The formation of a mature sperm takes about seventy days and can be likened to a conveyor-belt type of process. The sperm begins as a very basic cell and is constantly modified over those seventy days to become a cell that not only contains the male genetic information, but is also capable of actively seeking out and fertilizing an egg.

At the time of intercourse and ejaculation, the sperm move from the testicles through the vas deferens, through the urethra, and are deposited in the vagina. The sperm almost immediately begin to travel into the cervix and through the cervical mucus. The majority of sperm that reach the cervical mucus do so within a matter of just a few minutes. They then continue on into the uterus and up into the fallopian tubes. This is a long and arduous journey and has been likened in terms of relative length to a human swimming the English Channel back and forth seven times. Amazingly, the sperm can complete this journey in just a few minutes.

Of the millions of sperm deposited in the vagina, only a few hundred survive and make it into the fallopian tube—true survival of the fittest. The vast majority of the sperm in the ejaculate do not reach the cervical mucus and are killed in the acidic environment of the vagina. The ejaculate consists not only of the sperm but also of several cc's of fluid from the prostate, which nourishes and protects the sperm. Since only the sperm enter the cervix (and a very small percentage at that), it is normal for the majority of the ejaculate to "leak out" of the vagina following intercourse.

THE FEMALE AND THE EGGS

As opposed to the ongoing production of the sperm, new eggs are not formed within the ovaries. All of the eggs a woman will have, usually about two million, are present when she is born, and the number continues to decrease until, at the time of menopause, the egg supply is depleted. During each cycle many eggs begin to develop. Through a process that takes two to three weeks, usually just one of the eggs will reach maturity while the rest undergo a process known as atresia, or degeneration, and are lost forever. When that one egg is mature, it is released from the ovary and basically sits on the surface of the ovary surrounded by its protective cells. The egg will be capable of being fertilized for only the next twelve to maybe twenty-four hours at most. If not fertilized within that time, it is simply resorbed by the body.

FEMALE ANATOMY

The fallopian tube is the tube-like structure that sits between the uterus and ovary. The fimbria are lush, finger-like projections on the end of the tube near the ovary. When a mature egg is ovulated, the fimbria must actively seek out this egg and pick it up from the surface of the ovary; the egg does not just fall into the tube. Once the fimbria have picked up the egg, it is transported by little hair like projections on the surfaces of the cells on the inside of the tube toward the uterus into the portion of the tube known as the ampulla. It is here that the sperm and egg meet and that fertilization will occur. It doesn't take just one sperm to fertilize an egg. There are many protective cells surrounding the egg, and many sperm are lost while actively removing these cells in order to gain access to the egg. Only after these cells have been removed and a path cleared can a single sperm penetrate the egg. Once a sperm penetrates the egg, the protective layer around the egg immediately undergoes changes that prevent any further sperm from entering the egg.

After fertilization, the zygote, or early embryo, remains in the tube for another three or four days. While in the tube, continued development occurs. When the embryo is transported through the isthmic portion of the tube and into the uterus, it is usually about twenty to forty cells in size. The embryo "floats" in the uterus for an additional couple of days before attaching to the wall of the uterus, a process known as implantation.

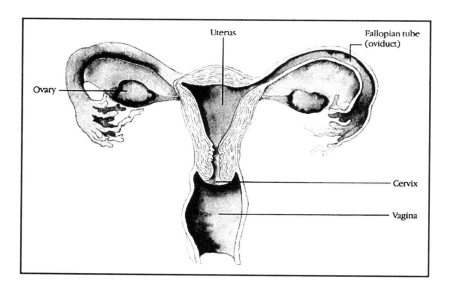

Timing Is Everything

There are very few days in the normal menstrual cycle during which a couple may conceive. While sperm may survive for several days in the reproductive tract of the female, the egg is only healthy and capable of being fertilized for twenty-four hours at most. After that time, it is simply resorbed by the body. The timing of this fertile period is, then, all determined by the process of egg development and ovulation. There are, really, only a few days at most during any given menstrual cycle during which conception can occur.

A normal menstrual cycle is defined as being twenty-eight to thirty days in length (from the start of one period to the start of the next). While cycles of shorter or longer length may or may not be normal, cycles of this length are most common. For purposes of discussion, Day 1 is defined as the first day of *normal* menstrual flow. During the next twelve to fourteen days, the events that result in the ovulation of a mature egg occur. This is called the "follicular phase," so called because the egg develops in a fluid-filled sac called the follicle. As the follicle (and the egg within it) develops, it produces hormones, the most important of which is estradiol (the primary form of estrogen).

Estradiol is responsible for stimulating other events to occur, all of which will result in optimal chances of the egg being fertilized and a pregnancy resulting. For example, estradiol is responsible for the changes in the cervical mucus. During much of the cycle, the cervical mucus is an impenetrable barrier, protecting the uterus and tubes from bacteria and anything else, including sperm. At about the time the egg is mature and ready to be released, the cervical mucus changes as a result of the ever increasing amounts of estradiol being produced by the follicle. The mucus becomes thin and watery, and rather than preventing sperm from entering the uterus, it actually enhances this activity for a couple of days (but only right around the time of ovulation). Estradiol is also responsible for the development of the lining of the uterus (the endometrium). All of these events occur in synchrony so that on day fourteen of the ideal twenty-eight-day cycle, ovulation occurs, the cervical mucus is penetrable, and the lining of the uterus is getting ready to accept an implantation.

Intercourse must occur reasonably near the time of ovulation. Shortly after ovulation, the cervical mucus again becomes too thick for the sperm to penetrate; too long before ovulation, the sperm simply will not survive long enough to fertilize the egg. Having intercourse every other day around the time of ovulation is probably optimal. If, for example, a couple has intercourse every other day (days ten, twelve, fourteen, and sixteen in a twenty-eight-day cycle), they have done all they can do—at least in terms of enhancing their chances of pregnancy. More frequent intercourse does not further improve the chances of pregnancy as there begins to be a decrease in the number of sperm available if intercourse occurs more frequently than once every forty-eight hours.

It is possible to predict ovulation, and thereby time intercourse. Ovulation is preceded by a surge, or rapid increase, of a hormone called LH (luteinizing hormone). This surge can be detected through the use of an ovulation predictor, which is an over-the-counter test sold in any drug store. There are many ovulation predictors available, but they all function by detecting an increase in the amount of LH in the urine. They are really quite reliable and may be of value in timing intercourse. When the ovulation predictor changes, suggesting imminent ovulation, it is time to have intercourse.

When Should We Worry?

The process is obviously more complex than outlined here, and each of these areas will be discussed in further detail in the appropriate chapter. These are, however, the basic steps in the process. The next question is "How well does this process normally work?" The answer is, "It depends." Human reproduction is a tremendously age-sensitive event. For a couple in their early twenties with no fertility problems, their fecundity, or chances of becoming pregnant in any given month, may be as high as twenty to twenty-five percent. This results in a probability of conception within one year of about ninety percent. For a couple in their forties with no known problems, monthly fecundity may be as low as one to two percent. These are important numbers to know. Numerous studies have demonstrated a significant decline in human fertility beginning at about age thirty and progressing rather quickly thereafter.

Many couples worry that it may be taking them too long to conceive. This is a natural concern. In this modern world, we are becoming ever more used to controlling anything and everything, and making things happen when we want. We can heat an entire meal in minutes or cross the country in hours. But we can't make ourselves be pregnant when we want. Nature doesn't work that way. Nature requires patience, and some couples have more patience than others.

The real question is this: "How long should a couple be patient before they begin to seek some help and evaluation?" The answer again is that "it depends." There are very specific definitions for the duration of unprotected intercourse before a couple should be considered infertile. A couple who has never been pregnant before is defined as infertile if they have been attempting pregnancy for one year without success. If a couple has a previous pregnancy but now have been trying for six months to have another child, they too are infertile by definition.

These are, however, only definitions. They do not mean that any couple must wait a mandatory year before they begin to seek some evaluation and help. In fact, in many cases, this wait would be inappropriate. Women beyond the age of thirty-five certainly should not wait a year before beginning at least some preliminary testing. After age forty, a good case can be made for suggesting that a couple contact a physician as soon as they make the decision to attempt pregnancy.

As a guideline, when a couple becomes concerned about their ability to conceive, they should schedule some time with a physician and talk it over. Depending on the circumstances, it may be that some simple reassurance is all that is warranted. It is, however, inappropriate for any physician to tell a couple "just relax, it will happen." If a couple is worried, their concerns need to be addressed. Equally inappropriate is the response, "You need to try for a year before we can do anything." This simply is not true. While it may not be appropriate to become overly concerned and perform a lot of expensive and extensive testing, some simple evaluation may go a long way toward reassurance. If a couple expresses fears and concerns, these emotions must be considered valid: To ignore or belittle them invalidates them, and this is not helpful or fair to anyone. So if you're worried, find a physician with an interest in fertility and schedule some time to talk to her or him. Just talking to someone about your concerns can't hurt.

You may or may not decide to pursue further testing at that time, but at least you can make that decision in a more informed fashion.

CHAPTER FIVE
GETTING STARTED

Once a couple decides they are concerned enough about their ability to conceive that they want to at least talk about it with a professional, the first step is to make an appointment with a physician. This doesn't necessarily have to be a specialist in fertility; many obstetrician-gynecologists and family practitioners are comfortable initiating a work-up. Sure, there are other things you can do. You can read a book; it may provide some useful information. You can talk to a friend, but be very careful! Sometimes the most well-intentioned advice from a friend such as "don't worry, just relax, it will happen" can hurt far more than anticipated and be worth just what you paid for it. And you can certainly continue to try on your own. But if you're worried, it will help to get some answers.

There is no substitute for a good history and physical exam. Every investigation into the cause of a couple's infertility must begin with a thorough history and physical. The physician is almost playing detective, looking for some information or a finding that will suggest a particular problem. Often a clue or clues will be discovered that can direct the initial investigation in a particular direction. No physician can begin to formulate the plan of evaluation appropriate for a couple until the physician becomes familiar with the perspective of the couple, taking a history of their attempts to conceive as well as of their general medical health, and doing a physical exam. *Remember: Not every couple needs every test. Evaluation must be tailored to the couple.*

One thing the physician needs to try to understand is "where the couple is coming from." How long have they been married? How long have they been trying to get pregnant? Have they used contraception in the past, and if so, what kind(s)? What, if any, evaluation have they had so far? How anxious are they? How frustrated are they? How aggressive do they want to be? How much do they feel that they can tolerate? The point is this: The approach for a twenty-five-year-old couple who have been trying for one year is going to be different than that for a thirty-eight-year-old woman and her forty-year-old husband who have been trying for three years.

EVALUATING THE MALE

The male should be questioned about his history. Has he ever fathered a child? Is there any history of trauma to the testes? Did he have mumps as an adult? Does he have any reason to believe that he may be subfertile? Has he had a prior semen analysis? Is there any history of infection? Is there any family history of infertility? The possibility of sexual dysfunction must also be explored. Is there any problem with maintaining an erection or with premature ejaculation? Does he ejaculate during intercourse? What is the frequency of sexual intercourse?

Semen Analysis

An initial semen analysis should almost always be ordered. Although it will undoubtedly produce some anxiety on the part of the husband, it has all of the characteristics of a test that should be ordered early; it is relatively easy, inexpensive, and noninvasive. And since up to forty percent of all infertility is related to some type of male factor, this is not a test that should be neglected.

Not all laboratories do semen analyses the same way. Try to find a lab that does a lot of semen analyses, or even better, one that specializes in semen analyses. If a specialized lab is not available, it's okay. Go ahead and get it done anyhow. It's too important to skip and any information is worthwhile.

Many specialists state that a male must have three semen analyses before anything can be said about the results. This is based on a couple of observations. First of all, producing a sample (masturbating) for a semen analysis for the first time can be rather unnerving. Often an initial sample will suggest a problem only to have later samples be perfectly normal. Secondly, sperm counts vary tremendously from day to day. If the first count is low, by all means repeat it. If the first count is normal, there is probably no need for three counts to confirm it.

Other Tests

Since most physicians specializing in infertility are obstetrician-gynecologists, or reproductive endocrinologists (obstetrician-gynecologists with specialty training), men are frequently not examined unless the initial semen analyses suggests that there is a problem. If the semen analysis is abnormal, the male may be referred to a urologist. The urologist will check the testes for abnormalities. They will also check for the presence of a varicocele, which is a dilated vein around the testes that can result in decreased sperm production. Some hormonal testing may also be ordered to try to discover the reason for decreased sperm production. Some urologists will recommend a testicular biopsy to further evaluate the problem, but there are very few, if any, cases in which a testicular biopsy will provide information that will allow improvement in a case of decreased sperm production. Be very certain why a testicular biopsy is being suggested and what the physician hopes to gain before undergoing this test.

Most importantly, the development of a procedure known as ICSI (see Intracytoplasmic Sperm Injection in Chapter 13) has changed much of the focus in the treatment of male infertility. Rather than trying to improve sperm production, much more success has been achieved by developing techniques that allow us to use what sperm are produced. In the past, attempts to increase sperm production have been disappointing at best. Recent developments such as ICSI have resulted in tremendous success, making fertilization and pregnancy with absolutely minimal numbers of sperm possible.

EVALUATING THE FEMALE

Female evaluation should also begin with a history and physical. Important aspects of the history include: 1) a complete gynecologic history, concentrating on the regularity and nature of the menstrual cycles, 2) a history of prior surgical procedures or pelvic infections, 3) prior pregnancies and the outcomes and complications thereof, 4) any dysmenorrhea, or pain with the periods, and the nature and history of that pain, and 5) the frequency of sexual intercourse, and any pain or problems associated therewith. A thorough history will also include a general medical history, including other illnesses or problems, smoking or drug use, and medications.

The physical exam should include an evaluation of the breasts, checking both for abnormalities and for discharge. A careful pelvic exam should also be performed. The ovaries and uterus can be carefully checked, with special attention to any findings that may suggest the presence of endometriosis (Chapter 9). A pelvic ultrasound is also worthwhile in that it allows the physician to see the ovaries and uterus and further ensures that no abnormalities are present.

Prolactin Level, Chlamydia Titer, and TSH

There should be no such thing as a "routine infertility panel" when it comes to blood tests. All testing should be individualized to the couple and dictated by the findings at the time of the history and physical. There are, however, a couple of tests that are almost always worthwhile: a prolactin level and a chlamydia titer. Prolactin is a pituitary hormone that controls breast milk production. It can be slightly to moderately elevated without causing any symptoms such as breast discharge. However, even slight elevations of prolactin can have significant effects on the menstrual cycles and thereby make it much harder if not impossible to conceive. *If cycles are anything but perfectly normal, prolactin should be checked.*

Chlamydia is an infectious organism that is sexually transmitted. Chlamydia can cause severe damage to the fallopian tubes without causing pain, fever or any other symptoms. The Centers for Disease Control considers chlamydia an epidemic. Therefore, since it is so widespread and since a woman may never know she has had it, this needs to be checked. A chlamydia culture can be performed which will detect an ongoing infection, but a better test is a chlamydia titer. A chlamydia titer is a blood test that will detect any prior exposure to chlamydia. If prior exposure is detected, and either partner is symptomatic or has a positive culture, both partners should be treated with a course of an appropriate antibiotic. This eliminates concerns about ongoing infection. As will be discussed later, the results of the chlamydia titer will dictate the procedure chosen for evaluation of the fallopian tubes.

Thyroid disturbances can also result in alterations of the menstrual cycles. TSH (thyroid-stimulating hormone) is the pituitary hormone that regulates the functioning of the thyroid gland. If the cycles are anything but perfectly normal, TSH should also be checked. If there is any abnormality of thyroid function, it will be reflected by this single test. An entire thyroid panel is necessary only if an abnormality of TSH is detected.

Ovulation

There are many ways to evaluate ovulation. The simplest of these is the basal body temperature (BBT) chart. This is an inexpensive, noninvasive, and relatively easy test. Using a specialized thermometer, the woman takes her temperature every morning before getting out of bed or doing anything, and then records it on a special chart.

BASAL BODY TEMPERATURE CHART
(see reverse for instructions)

Name _____

Date of Birth _____

Basal Body Temperature Chart

If BBTs are recorded for a couple of months, they will provide the physician with important information about the cycles. BBTs will demonstrate clearly not only the length of the cycles, and their regularity, but also the approximate time of ovulation and the length of the second half of the cycle.

There are several aspects of BBTs that are important to remember:

1. Don't try to interpret them yourself, especially day to day. It will drive you crazy trying to make sense of the changes. Temperature charts really only make sense when looked at in terms of the entire cycle.

2. Don't use temperatures to predict ovulation. The temperature goes up after you ovulate—once the temperature goes up it is too late to have intercourse in hopes of getting pregnant. You may hear that there is a drop in the temperature at the time of ovulation and that this can be used to time intercourse. Well, sometimes there is and sometimes there isn't, but it certainly isn't reliable enough to use to time intercourse. (Ovulation predictors work much better.)

3. Don't record BBTs for too long. A couple of cycles is usually enough unless the physician wants to evaluate the response to a change in medications. Infertility is difficult enough—the last thing you need is a daily reminder in the form of a thermometer in your mouth the first thing when you wake up every morning.

4. If you forget a couple of days, don't worry. Just record as many days as you can.

5. Record any information on the chart you think may be worthwhile.

6. After a couple of months, sit down with your physician and review the charts.

There are also many brands of ovulation predictors sold over the counter. Most of these are very simple to perform, one-step tests that you do at home. All of these tests function by identifying large amounts of the hormone LH in the urine. (LH is the trigger of ovulation and rises significantly twenty-four to thirty-six hours before ovulation.) These are reliable tests and are good predictors of ovulation. They can be helpful not only for timing intercourse, but also for providing additional information when coupled with a BBT chart.

The Postcoital Test

The cervical mucus thins out just prior to ovulation and actually facilitates the transfer of the sperm to the uterus. The postcoital test (PCT) is a good way to evaluate not only the cervical mucus, but also the interaction of the sperm and the mucus. This test must be performed right around the time of ovulation. It cannot be performed more than a couple of days before ovulation, nor after ovulation, as the cervical mucus will be too thick for this test to be meaningful.

Following intercourse, a sample of cervical mucus is gently removed from the cervix at the time of a normal pelvic exam and evaluated microscopically. The quality of the cervical mucus as well as the number of sperm present and their motility can all be checked. While it is often stated that this test must be performed within two hours of intercourse, it can actually be checked as many as twelve to fourteen hours after intercourse (do not douche or take a bath, but showers are okay) as long as the physician is informed of the time. If properly timed, this test reveals a great deal about the adequacy of the cervical mucus production, the survivability of the sperm in the cervical mucus, and the interaction of the sperm and the cervical mucus.

Evaluating The Fallopian Tubes

There are basically two techniques available for evaluating the fallopian tubes: a hysterosalpingogram and a laparoscopy.

Hysterosalpingogram (HSG)

A hysterosalpingogram (HSG) is an X-ray procedure that does not require any anesthesia and can be performed in just a few minutes. It is performed at the time in the cycle after the period stops but before ovulation occurs. A regular speculum exam is performed in the X-ray department, and a small instrument is attached to the cervix. A special X-ray dye is then injected through the cervix, up into the uterus, and out into the fallopian tubes. This procedure allows visualization of the uterine cavity and of the fallopian tubes. If the tubes are open, the dye can be seen spilling into the abdominal cavity.

The advantages of the HSG include the fact that it is a nonsurgical procedure, does not require anesthesia, and is relatively inexpensive. *A further advantage is the fact that if oil-soluble dye is used, pregnancy rates after a HSG are actually increased, thus rendering it therapeutic as well as diagnostic.* (HSG can be performed using water-soluble contrast material or oil-soluble contrast material; postprocedure enhancement of conception rates has been demonstrated only following the use of oil-soluble contrast material.) The biggest disadvantage of the HSG is the inability to visualize other pelvic structures. Only the interior of the tubes and uterus can be seen, and thus adhesions, endometriosis, or other problems lying outside the tubes and uterine cavity may go undetected.

Laparoscopy

Laparoscopy is an outpatient surgical procedure performed under general anesthesia, although microinstruments are now available that allow this procedure to also be performed in the office under local anesthesia. A small telescopelike instrument is inserted into the abdominal cavity just beneath the umbilicus (navel). This allows visualization of the abdominal contents in their entirety, including the ovaries, tubes, uterus and the surrounding structures. Additional small incisions may be placed in the abdominal wall to allow insertion of specially designed instruments, including lasers.

Laparoscopy does not need to be a purely diagnostic procedure. Many physicians performing laparoscopic surgery have the ability to correct virtually any abnormality that they may encounter. Laparoscopy should probably be done each and every time as a potentially operative and therapeutic procedure. Find out if your physician has the ability to treat endometriosis, remove adhesions, correct tubal blockage and remove ovarian cysts through the laparoscope. Some surgeons prefer to do laparoscopy as a purely diagnostic procedure and then do major surgery to correct abnormalities they may encounter. While both approaches are equally effective, the latter has the disadvantage of requiring two surgeries and being significantly more expensive.

The biggest advantage of laparoscopy over the HSG is its potential for surgical correction of abnormalities. It does also allow direct visualization of the abdominal contents. The disadvantages of laparoscopy include the fact that it is invasive, requires general anesthesia, and is vastly more expensive than an HSG.

The decision as to which of these procedures should be used to evaluate the tubes must again be based on the individual circumstances. The findings on a pelvic exam must be considered. If there is significant, palpable endometriosis, or especially if ovarian endometriosis is noted on ultrasound, then laparoscopy may be indicated. Similarly, if the chlamydia titer is high suggesting prior infection, if there is a history of prior infection, or if there has been previous pelvic surgery, then laparoscopy must be considered. Note that these are all specific indications for proceeding with a laparoscopy. *There should be a very specific reason for choosing laparoscopy over HSG. If there is not some specific indication for doing a laparoscopy, then the HSG is the procedure of choice for tubal evaluation.*

In the following chapters, we will look at each step in the evaluation process in more detail and begin to see how these steps suggest which interventions may be worthwhile. The evaluation process must always be dynamic and ongoing. In up to forty percent of couples, more than one factor contributes to their difficulty conceiving. *It should not be presumed that because one factor has been discovered there may not be another factor that may be equally or more important.*

CHAPTER SIX
CHANCES ARE

Since ancient times, there have been gods, magical potions, and special spells for helping with fertility. The ancient Mayans prayed to the fertility god Quetzalcoatl to restore their fertility. And it worked! There are, after all, relatively few problems that render a couple absolutely incapable of conceiving. Most of the time a couple's fertility is compromised, but not absolutely. We all know stories of couples who have given up their attempts to get pregnant only to conceive shortly thereafter. Or couples who have adopted one child and all of a sudden they conceive and have two children under the age of two. This is not to imply that giving up, or adopting, increases one's chances of conceiving. It doesn't! The point is this: Every treatment, be it praying to Quetzalcoatl, trying on your own without intervention, or pursuing the most high-tech options available has a certain chance of being successful each month or with each attempt.

Finding exact numbers for your chances of getting pregnant within any given time frame can be one of the most frustrating aspects of trying to get pregnant. This chapter will examine the considerations involved in trying to decide what should be done, and when it should be done.

AGE AND DURATION OF ATTEMPTS

The first consideration must always be, "what are the chances if we just keep trying on our own?" Fecundity, or the likelihood of getting pregnant each month, is tremendously age dependent. For a couple in their early twenties with no known problems, fecundity may be as high as twenty to twenty-five percent per cycle. For a couple in their early forties with no known problems this number is less than five percent. There is clearly a decline in fertility beginning at about age thirty. This becomes more dramatic after age thirty-five, and after age forty, it is very significant. This decline in a couple's chances of getting pregnant each month must be coupled with miscarriage rates that clearly increase as a woman gets older, ranging from about eighteen percent in younger couples to as high as twenty-five to fifty percent in women over age forty. Just on the basis of this information, a more conservative approach to fertility treatment is often justified in younger couples, whereas a more aggressive approach may be more appropriate for an older couple.

How long a couple has been trying to conceive is also important. The definitions of infertility suggest that a couple is not infertile unless they having been trying for a year to conceive their first pregnancy, or until they have been trying for six months after having been pregnant before. These are only definitions. They don't mean that if you have been trying for a year your chances for the next month become zero. While statistically the chances may be decreased enough that some evaluation may be warranted, they may still be very real. But, at the same time, it is clear that the longer a couple has been trying, the less likely it is that they will be successful. Data clearly show that a couple's fecundity decreases in direct proportion to the length of time they have been trying to conceive. In other words, if a couple has been trying to conceive for five years, their chances of conceiving in the next month probably are not zero, but they certainly aren't very good.

MEDICAL CONSIDERATIONS

Age and duration of attempts are very important considerations, not only in deciding when to seek help, but also in tailoring an evaluation and treatment plan that is appropriate for each individual couple. And once an investigation is begun, so are the results of that investigation. Physicians use the information they gather to try and formulate an equation that will give them some idea of what each individual couple's chances are without intervention, and what they would be with any given type of intervention. The semen analysis and any identified female factors must be taken into account, and reasonable treatment alternatives determined.

There are very few couples in whom infertility is absolute. Complete absence of sperm (azoospermia), total tubal occlusion and ovarian failure are the exceptions. In couples with these particular problems, determining treatment options is relatively straightforward. In couples without absolute infertility, determining appropriate options can be much more difficult. There are a couple of "factors of discrimination" that are helpful. The first is the semen analysis. The number of functional sperm is one factor that dictates which options are reasonable. If there are thirty million normal sperm present, many alternatives, from conservative to aggressive, may be reasonable. If, on the other hand, the semen analysis shows only one million sperm with very poor motility, anything but ICSI may have virtually no chance of success. The second is the status of the fallopian tubes. As long as we know the tubes are open and appear normal, many approaches may be reasonable. If they are occluded or damaged, IVF may be the only choice with a realistic chance of success.

The physician's task, then, is to consider this information, these factors of discrimination, as well as all the other data gathered. The number of factors identified that may be contributing to a couple's inability to conceive is very important. If a couple has more than one infertility factor, the effect of each factor on their infertility is not additive. It is almost exponential! The number of identified infertility factors is an extremely important consideration.

The physician must, then, consider:
1. The couple's age, particularly that of the female
2. The length of time a couple has been infertile
3. What problems have been identified and
4. How many problems have been identified.

Based on these considerations, the physician must decide what he or she thinks are reasonable treatment alternatives. The physician should then be able to say to a couple:

"This is alternative A. Here is what is involved in pursuing alternative A. Here is what it will cost to pursue alternative A. And these are your chances of success per attempt with this approach"; and

"This is alternative B. Here is what is involved in pursuing alternative B. Here is what it will cost to pursue alternative B. And these are your chances of success per attempt with this approach."

For example, what are the alternatives for John and Mary, both aged thirty-five, who have been trying for three years to conceive? Their evaluation has been entirely normal.

1. Continue trying without intervention. (The chances probably aren't zero, but after three years of trying at age thirty-five, they are getting pretty small.)

2. Try clomiphene. (They were on clomiphene for six months with a prior physician. The chances of being successful in a seventh cycle of clomiphene don't justify its use.)

3. Superovulation with gonadotropins ± inseminations (Chapter 12).

4. An ART procedure (Chapter 13).

The last two alternatives seem to be the only ones that are reasonable. Now what John and Mary need is as much information about those two alternatives as they can get. It is the physician's job to determine which options are reasonable and to provide the couple with all pertinent information concerning those options. *It is the couple's job to decide what they want to do! All decisions must be made by the physician and the couple as a team.*

PERSONAL CONSIDERATIONS

Only the couple can take the information the physician has provided and evaluate it in terms of their life situation. Real-world constraints and considerations are extremely important in this whole process. Some of the "real-world factors" that must be considered include:

Work

Very few women in this day and age have the luxury of being able to devote all of their time to trying to get pregnant. They have to pursue their careers at the same time. How much time away from work will each alternative require, and how much can you afford? Can you pursue an alternative and still work? Some women even schedule certain treatments during vacations.

Stress Levels

The stress associated with infertility is second only to the stress associated with the death of a loved one! How much of a toll has that stress already taken on you, your self-esteem, your marriage? How much more can you tolerate? For example: Given two alternatives, a couple who has been trying to conceive for five years may decide to pursue the alternative with the best per-attempt chance of success simply because they just can't tolerate a whole lot more.

One inexorable force couples face as they pursue fertility is the "ticking of the biological clock," making it seem as if their efforts are taking forever. It can make you feel old long before you should. This clock is often every bit as much an enemy as it is an ally. It makes every cycle that ends with a menstrual period that much harder to tolerate. And it can make couples do silly things out of desperation. Don't ever do something just to be doing something. *Make sure the options you pursue are reasonable and offer you a decent chance of success.*

Geography

Fertility services are not available everywhere. If you have to travel several hundred miles, your choice of alternatives might tend to be more aggressive than it would be if you only have to go across the street.

Cost

Insurance coverage for fertility services is extremely variable. Medications, testing, procedures, etc. may or may not be covered. And fertility services can be expensive. The cost/success ratio of each alternative must be a consideration.

DECIDING ON A TREATMENT

A couple needs to be well informed by their physician regarding their reasonable treatment alternatives. And they have to be in touch with their perspective in order to decide which of those alternatives they are most comfortable pursuing. If your physician evaluates your particular case and provides you with reasonable information concerning your alternatives, and if you decide between these alternatives within the framework of your real-world factors, then there are no wrong decisions. You can't make a bad choice!

But you and your physician must constantly reevaluate. Each and every form of therapy, from praying to Quetzalcoatl to attempting in vitro fertilization, has a cumulative success curve that will "flatten out" after a given number of attempts. In other words, if you have tried one approach for several cycles and it hasn't worked, the chances that it will work in the next cycle begin to diminish. And after a certain length of time, that approach may not increase your chances at all. *Any approach should be pursued only as long as it is clearly keeping you on the steep part of the cumulative success curve.*

Hypothetical Cumulative Success Curves

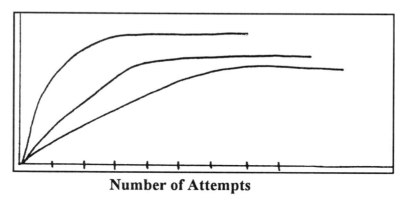

Percent Pregnant

Number of Attempts

These lines represent theoretical cumulative success curves for various forms of therapy. Every form of therapy or treatment has a cumulative success curve that will "flatten out" after a given number of attempts. No therapy should be pursued into the flat part of the curve.

If, after a given while a certain choice is unsuccessful, talk it over again with your physician, examine your alternatives and decide what you should do next. Communication is key, and proper decision making requires a partnership between you and your physician. An informed, well-thought-out decision can't be wrong.

And don't hesitate to take breaks. Many couples feel that if they take some time off and stop concentrating on trying to conceive for a while, they are being negligent and their chances will be that much less when they do start trying again. This just isn't so! Infertility is very stressful, and there is no doubt that the stress can take its toll. Breaks, or treatment vacations, are wonderful ideas. They restore the emotional energy required to pursue treatment and deal with the results. They also remind a couple that intercourse is something that can be done for fun rather than just on certain days at certain times. Don't hesitate to take breaks. They are good for the soul!

REACHING RESOLUTION

The obvious goal of every physician who treats couples with infertility is to help each and every one of them conceive. This is an unattainable goal. While the *vast majority* of couples with infertility can be helped, and do conceive, there still exists a certain percentage who never will conceive. *A much more realistic goal would be to help each and every couple reach resolution.* The more couples for which this means pregnancy, the better. But those couples who don't conceive need to reach resolution as well. When all available alternatives have been attempted, and when they have been attempted enough times that the success curve is flat, the physician must be willing to inform a couple of this. The physician must be willing to inform a couple when they have exhausted all reasonable treatment options. And when a couple feels they have given it their all, when they feel good about their efforts and can look themselves in the mirror and say "we did all we could do," they have reached resolution. Achieving pregnancy for every couple is a very lofty goal indeed. Achieving resolution for every couple is what the job is all about.

CHAPTER SEVEN
THE MALE FACTOR

SEMEN ANALYSIS

Difficulty conceiving is related to some compromise of the sperm count or sperm function in as many as forty percent of all couples. Therefore, *a semen analysis should be one of the very first tests done.* A semen analysis is easy (ignoring the embarrassment some men may feel), inexpensive and noninvasive. Evaluation of the sperm is a point of discrimination: The sperm count will dictate which options are reasonable for a couple to pursue in their attempts to conceive. A severely compromised sperm count may, for example, mean that only rather sophisticated procedures are worthwhile, whereas a normal count would allow consideration of much more conservative procedures.

Obtaining and Delivering the Sample

A semen sample is usually obtained by masturbation with collection of the ejaculate into a sterile specimen container. No lubricants should be used. There are also specially designed condoms that can be worn during intercourse to collect a semen sample. (These do have to be special condoms, which are available through your physician.) Two to three days of abstinence is suggested before obtaining a sample for analysis. Longer periods of abstinence may increase the count, but the percentage of sperm that are actively motile will decrease. Conversely, shorter periods of abstinence may result in some decrease in the number of sperm present. Two to three days of abstinence before a semen analysis provides the most accurate results.

The sample should be submitted for analysis as soon as possible after collection. It is preferable to collect the sample at the office or laboratory where the analysis will be performed. Specially designed rooms just for this purpose are usually available. If you are going to collect the sample at home, keep it at body temperature while transporting it to the laboratory. Placing the container under your arm, inside your pants, or in your bra will accomplish this. The sooner the sample is provided to the laboratory after collection the better.

Interpreting Semen Reports

Examples of two reports of semen analysis results are provided below. It is easy to see that there is much more detailed information available in the second report.

The first is a report fairly typical of a laboratory that does not really specialize in evaluating semen samples.

Clinical Laboratory - Community General Hospital
Any City

Date: _____   Patient Name: _____
SS#: _____   Physician: _____

Test	Result	Expected Range	Units
Semen analysis - Fertility			
Semen Volume	2.5	2.0 - 5.0	mL
Sperm Motility	65	60-100	%
Sperm Count	89	60-150	M/mL

There is nothing wrong with this type of analysis, and often for a first test, this is fine. If it is perfectly normal, it's probably pretty reliable but this information is obviously limited. If there is any question at all about the normalcy of the results from this type of laboratory, the second test should be done by a laboratory that can do a more detailed analysis.

There is obviously far more information and detail provided by the second sperm analysis. This test was analyzed by a laboratory that specializes in evaluating sperm samples. Following is an explanation of the information obtained and what the results mean.

Indianapolis Andrology & Laboratory Services, Inc.

Semen Analysis & Medical History

Specimen Date _____   Date of Birth _____

Husband Name _____   Husband S.S. # _____

Address _____   Wife Name _____

City/State/Zip Code _____   Home Phone (   ) _____

Referring Physician _____   Work Phone (   ) _____

Days of Abstinence _____ Post Vasectomy: Yes _____ No _____   Method of Collection: _____

Specimen I.D. #_____

INITIAL
SEMEN ANALYSIS: Time Collected _____ Time Submitted _____ Time Evaluated _____

Coagulum Present _____ Yes _____ No   Liquified in: _____ 30 _____ 60 _____ 90 minutes

Volume _____ml   Normal: 2.0 ml or more

Viscosity: High   1 _____   2 _____   3 _____   4 _____ low

Motility: A. % Rapid Progression _____

             B. % Slow Progression_____

             C. % Non-Progressive _____

             D. % Immotile_____

NORMAL: > 25% "a" pattern or > 50% "a+b" pattern

Viability: _____% Normal: > 75%

Sperm Agglutination: Slight _____ Moderate _____ Heavy _____

Sperm Aggregation: Slight _____ Moderate _____ Heavy _____

pH _____ Normal: 7.2 – 8.0

Sperm Concentration: _____ Normal: 20×10^6/ml

Total Count: _____ Normal: 40×10^6

Fructose _____ mg   Normal > 2.4mg/ejaculation

Leukocyte Concentration _____ 1×10^6/ml

Total motile normal sperm _____

BLOOD HORMONE LEVELS	**Male Normal Ranges**
DHEA-SO_4 _____	80 - 560 ug/dl
Estradiol _____	6 - 44 pg/ml
FSH_____	2 - 9 mIU/ml
HCG _____	< 1.0 mIU/ml
LH _____	0.4 - 3.7 mIU/ml
Progesterone _____	0.0 - 0.4 ng/ml
Prolactin _____	3 - 17 ng/ml
Testosterone_____	270 - 1070 ng/dl
T_3U _____%	25 - 35%
T_4 _____	4.5 - 12.5 ug/dl
T_7 _____	3.6 - 14.9
TSH_____	2-20 Yrs. 0.7 - 5.7 21-54 Yrs. 0.4-4.2 54-87 Yrs. 0.5-8.9

Morphology %	Normal Sperm	Slightly Amorphous	Severely Amorphous	Midpiece/Tail Defect	Immature Cells	NORMAL: >4% Normal or >30% Normal and slightly amorphous

Comments: _____

_____

_____

Jeffrey P. Boldt, Ph.D
Laboratory Director

TECH:_____ DATE:_____

8081 Township Line Road, Indianapolis, IN 46260 • (317) 875-5978 • (800) 333-1415

MEDICAL HISTORY

1. a) Age _____ yrs.   b) Wife/Partner's Age _____ yrs.

2. Period of Unprotected Intercourse: _____ yrs.

   Prior contraceptive methods:

   a) ____ None   b) ____ Diaphragm   c) ____ IUD   d) ____ Pill   e) ____ Vasectomy   f) ____Tubal Ligation

3. Have you ever fathered a child by: a) Current Partner: _____ Yes   _____ No

                                          b) Other Partner: _____ Yes   _____ No

   Has your wife had a child / been pregnant by: a) Yourself   _____ Yes   _____ No

                                                     b) Other Partner: _____ Yes   _____ No

4. Frequency of Intercourse: _____ per week   _____ per month

5. Loss of sexual desire: _____ Yes   _____ No

6. Any problems with erections: _____ Yes   _____ No

7. Any problem with ejaculation: _____ Yes   _____ No   _____ Premature   _____ Delayed

                                  _____ Retrograde (feeling but without forward ejaculation from penis)

8. Delayed testicular descent into scrotum: _____ Yes   _____ No

   If yes, was corrective surgery performed: _____ Yes (at age _____ years)   _____ No

9. Any history of testicular injury: _____ Yes   _____ No   Mumps: _____ Yes   _____ No

   Sport Injury: _____ Yes   _____ No   Approx. age when disease occurred: _____

10. High Blood Pressure: ____ Yes   _____ No

    What medications (if any) for high blood pressure? _____

11. Peptic Ulcer: _____ Yes   _____ No

    Medication for peptic ulcer: _____ Tagamet   _____ Zantac   Other _____

12. Respiratory Infections: _____ Yes   _____ No

13. Cancer: _____ Yes   _____ No

    If yes, how treated: _____ Surgery   _____ Radiation   _____ Chemotherapy

14. Lameness or weakness in buttocks or legs, relieved by rest: _____ Yes   _____ No

15. Diabetes Mellitus: _____ Yes   _____ No   Insulin: _____ Yes   _____ No

16. Recreational Drugs: _____ Alcohol   _____ Smoking   _____ Marijuana

17. Heavy exercise: _____ Yes   _____No   Anabolic Steroids: _____ Yes   _____ No

    Hot Tubs: _____ Yes   _____ No

Comments: _____

_____

_____

_____

Coagulum present: The ejaculate normally "coagulates" into a jellylike blob within a few minutes of ejaculation.

Liquefied in: The coagulum should begin to break down and liquefy within thirty to sixty minutes of ejaculation.

Volume: Two to four cc's is normal. Larger or smaller volumes may present a problem in getting enough sperm to the cervix either because there is not enough seminal fluid to protect the sperm in the vagina or because the sperm present are diluted in too large a volume.

Viscosity: This is a measure of the overall stickiness of the sample.

Motility: This is the measure of the rate at which the sperm move. Good sperm motility is vital to their ability to fertilize an egg. Only those sperm with rapid progression can reach and fertilize an egg. Sperm may also be slowly progressive (moving, but not moving well, or moving in very erratic patterns), nonprogressive (alive and shaking, literally, but not moving), and immotile (alive but not moving at all). Some distinction about grade of motility is important and sometimes missing from more cursory evaluations.

Viability: The percentage that are alive regardless of their motility.

Agglutination and aggregation: Measures of the extent to which the sperm are stuck to each other or stuck to material within the ejaculate.

pH: The pH of the seminal fluid must be within the range of 7.2 to 8.0 to protect the sperm from the very acidic environment of the vagina until they can reach the cervix.

Sperm concentration: The number of sperm present in one cc.

Total count: The sperm concentration multiplied by the volume.

Fructose: Fructose is the sugar present in the seminal fluid. It functions as an energy source for the sperm and is produced in the seminal vesicle.

Absence of fructose suggests an obstruction in the path of the sperm from the testicles to the penis.

Leukocyte concentration: Leukocytes are white blood cells, and their presence suggests an infection, often of the prostate gland. This is reported as the number of white cells per 100 sperm present.

Morphology: This is the microscopic assessment of the appearance of the sperm. There are two techniques for evaluating morphology. The "standard technique" is done much more superficially and with this technique, most laboratories use sixty percent normal sperm as their cut-off point for a normal semen analysis. The second technique uses the "strict criteria." With this technique, the sperm are much more critically assessed, and a sperm must be perfectly normal to be so considered. Under these criteria, more than fourteen percent normal-appearing sperm is outstanding, and more than four percent is probably normal. The use of the "strict criteria" for evaluating morphology is validated by the good correlation between normal appearance by these criteria and the fertilizing capacity of a sperm. Most labs specializing in semen analyses will use the "strict" criteria.

Total motile normal sperm (also known as TMNS):This is the "bottom line" of the semen analysis. This is the number of sperm that are normal by strict criteria and possess rapid progressive motility. In other words, this is how many sperm in the sample are capable of fertilizing an egg. The TMNS provides the physician with a number that he or she can use to determine which treatment alternatives will offer a couple an acceptable chance of conception.

OTHER TESTS OF SPERM FUNCTION

Sperm penetration assay: A test in which sperm are incubated with specially prepared hamster eggs (actual fertilization cannot occur). The ability of the sperm to bind to the eggs and penetrate them is measured. The results of this test correlate moderately well with the ability to penetrate a human egg: If there is good penetration in this assay, there is a very good chance the sperm are capable of penetrating a human egg.

Sperm antibody tests: These tests check for the production of antibodies by either the male or female. Antibodies are substances that can either immobilize or even kill the sperm before the sperm can reach the egg. In order to detect antibodies, a tube of blood is drawn from the woman and incubated with a sperm sample in the laboratory and examined microscopically.

Mannose test, acrosome reaction test: Before a sperm can attach to and fertilize an egg, it must undergo a process known as capacitation. Capacitation involves changes in the membrane of the head of the sperm that are necessary to allow attachment to, and penetration of, the egg. These tests measure the ability of the sperm to undergo capacitation and allow identification of sperm that may not be able to fertilize an egg in spite of an otherwise normal semen analysis. These tests can be particularly useful in cases of unexplained infertility or prior to an ART procedure. These are also known as sperm function tests (SFTs).

Sperm washing or Percoll gradient: Techniques used to isolate the healthiest and most motile sperm. A semen sample is subjected to one of these procedures prior to, for example, inseminations.

Testicular biopsy: A technique in which a small piece of the testicle(s) is surgically removed and microscopically evaluated. The value of this procedure in terms of suggesting ways to improve the sperm count is questionable at best. With the availability of microinsemination techniques such as ICSI (intracytoplasmic sperm injection), a testicular biopsy may be worthwhile in that if it demonstrates the presence of even a few very immature sperm, these can now be used to achieve fertilization and pregnancies.

CAUSES OF ABNORMAL SPERM COUNTS

Heat: Sperm production is sensitive to heat—so sensitive, in fact, that placing the testicles at normal body temperature on a chronic basis stops sperm production altogether. The temperature in the testicles is about four degrees lower than body temperature. Anything that tends to keep the temperature in the testicles elevated for long periods of time will likewise have a negative effect. Excessive use of hot tubs or saunas or maybe even prolonged and heavy exercise may decrease sperm production and motility. One example often cited of an occupational exposure to excessive heat is truck drivers or farmers who often work long, hot hours in heavy clothing such as blue jeans.

Cigarettes, Alcohol, and Nonprescription Drugs: Cigarette smoking and alcohol abuse adversely affect sperm counts and sperm function. This is not to imply that having a beer or two on the weekend needs to be avoided, but significant alcohol intake can have a very significant effect. In short, if you drink, do so in moderation. If you smoke, QUIT.

Illicit drugs definitely affect sperm counts. Marijuana and cocaine are the prime examples of drugs that interfere with sperm production. Anabolic steroid use is also well known to decrease sperm production.

Prescription Drugs, Infections and Illnesses: Certain medications may also have a negative effect. Sulfasalazine (used for ulcerative colitis), cimetidine (used for ulcers), and calcium-channel blockers (used for high blood pressure) alter sperm production and function. The use of any medication on a chronic basis should be brought to the attention of your physician. Prenatal exposure to DES (diethylstilbestrol, a hormone used in the past to help prevent miscarriage) can dramatically decrease sperm production.

Certain infections, such as mumps contracted after puberty, have been clearly shown to dramatically affect sperm counts. Others, such as the presence of white cells in a semen analysis in a man who is otherwise asymptomatic are less clear, but treatment is probably indicated and may result in some improvement.

Chronic illnesses, such as diabetes, are important. Prior treatment for cancer by surgery, radiation or chemotherapy can also be significant.

Other causes: Obviously, a history of a prior vasectomy is important. There may be increased antibody production in men who have had a prior vasectomy and a reversal. The same may be true in individuals who have experienced significant injuries to the testicles.

Finally, does chronic stress have a negative impact? Maybe! Long-term, high-stress situations can lead to a decrease in testosterone production, and possibly in sperm production.

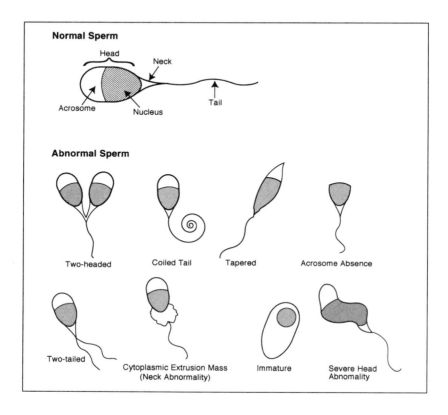

Normal Sperm

Head
Neck
Acrosome
Nucleus
Tail

Abnormal Sperm

Two-headed | Coiled Tail | Tapered | Acrosome Absence

Two-tailed | Cytoplasmic Extrusion Mass (Neck Abnormality) | Immature | Severe Head Abnomality

TREATMENT OPTIONS FOR SPERM PROBLEMS

There are ways to improve sperm counts, and we will detail those in the next few paragraphs. However, the treatment of male infertility and improvement of sperm counts has been a frustrating problem for both the patient and the physician for a long time. The process of spermatogenesis is an extremely complex one that occurs over the course of about seventy days. Our understanding of this remarkable process is rudimentary, at best, and our ability to define where a problem exists and to correct it is almost nonexistent. Until recently, we could do nothing for many cases. Now, however, with the advent of laboratory techniques such as IVF and ICSI, we have the ability to take the most compromised of sperm samples and achieve fertilization in the laboratory. Men with even just a few sperm *can* achieve pregnancy. The bottom line when it comes to treating male fertility is this: Much of the focus in the treatment of male infertility has shifted from trying to improve sperm production and quality to finding ways to work with whatever sperm are present.

Schedule Wisely

It's important to realize that it takes about seventy days for the testicles to produce a sperm that is fully mature and ready to achieve fertilization. Any significant insult during that seventy-day period can significantly affect the sperm count for two to three months. For example, if you have a very high fever today as the result of the flu or an infection, it may be three months before your sperm count will fully return to normal. Keep this in mind when scheduling your sperm counts—if you have any reason to think there may have been some event that could interfere with sperm production, it may be wise to wait a while between sperm counts and see if the count improves.

Remember to avoid toxins—it's that simple. You don't necessarily have to abstain from drinking alcohol, but be reasonable. And, if there is any evidence of infection, treat it. It's straightforward, inexpensive, non-invasive, and it may help.

Urologist Evaluation

Evaluation by a urologist, particularly one who has a special interest in male fertility, is usually the first step in evaluating abnormal semen analyses. There are several problems that urologists treat effectively.

1. Varicocele: A varicocele is a dilated vein or veins around the testicles. It is thought that these dilated veins increase the heat of the testicle and thereby impair sperm production and the motility of the sperm that are produced. This effect of a varicocele can be progressive over time. Significant varicoceles can usually be appreciated on a simple physical exam. Correction of a varicocele requires a minor surgical procedure and can result in dramatic improvements in sperm numbers and function if the varicocele is large. Smaller varicoceles may or may not be important, and

correction of small varicoceles is not likely to result in clinically significant improvements in the sperm count.

2. Obstruction: Most obstructions of the male reproductive tract are due to prior vasectomies, although they may occur as a result of infection, prior surgery (e.g., hernia repair), or may even be congenital. Microsurgery in the hands of one experienced in this technique can be very successful in reversing obstruction. The chances of successfully reversing an obstruction decrease the longer the obstruction has been present.

3. Failure of ejaculation: There are medications available that can remedy this problem for a large number of individuals. In others (for example, men who have suffered a spinal cord injury) electroejaculation has been very successful.

4. Retrograde ejaculation: In some individuals, the sperm are actually ejaculated backward into the bladder rather than out through the penis. This can be a congenital abnormality, or it may occur as the result of surgery, illness (*e.g.,* diabetes) or medications. This can often be corrected through the use of medications, but if this does not work, the sperm can be isolated from the urine and used for insemination.

5. Testicular cooling: The testicles don't work well if they are too hot. Taking steps to keep the testicles cool is a very reasonable thing to do. Wear boxer shorts instead of jockey shorts. Avoid long or frequent saunas or hot tubs. Sleep naked. Finally, there is some suggestion that actually placing a small ice pack in a sock and then sitting on it for a while in the evening may be worthwhile.

Medical Therapies

Clomiphene citrate (Clomid, Serophene): Clomiphene citrate is an orally administered medication often used in women because it leads to an increased production of FSH by the pituitary, stimulating the ovaries. The rationale behind the use of clomiphene in men is that it will result in increased levels of FSH stimulating the testicles to produce more sperm. There is no good evidence that the use of clomiphene in men results in improved sperm production or better pregnancy rates.

Human menopausal gonadotropins: These medications are actually preparations of the hormones FSH and LH (Pergonal, Humegon), or FSH alone (Metrodin, Fertinex, Gonal-F, Follistim). They must be administered by injections, usually on a daily basis, and they are very expensive. In the rare individual whose pituitary does not produce LH and FSH, these preparations can be quite effective. In individuals whose pituitary gland functions normally but the sperm count is decreased, the value of these medications is much more questionable.

Human chorionic gonadotropin (hCG): Although this was a popular form of therapy in the past, it has not been found to be of value and is rarely used anymore.

Vitamins: There have been reports touting everything from vitamin E to vitamin C to zinc as the cure for decreased sperm production. I would suggest that everyone take some nice multivitamin, not megadoses, and leave it at that.

THE MALE ALGORITHM

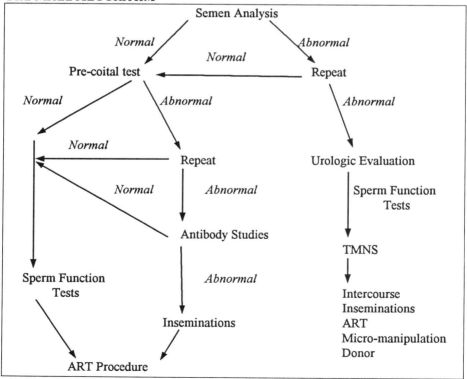

This chart demonstrates the algorithm for the evaluation and management of the male. It will allow a couple to understand the steps involved and follow along with the evaluation. This same chart is reproduced in the back of the book in a form that allows a couple to record and chart the findings as they are obtained.

SEMEN ANALYSIS

Semen analyses were discussed in detail above. If the semen analysis is abnormal, it should be repeated. Before repeating it, eliminate any of the possible causes of abnormal evaluations as listed above. Also be sure to repeat it after an adequate period of time has elapsed to allow improvement to occur. Remember, it takes seventy days to produce a mature sperm.

Postcoital Test

If the semen analysis is normal, the next step should be a post-coital test. The postcoital test (also known as the Huhner Test) is an excellent means of assessing the interaction of the sperm and the cervical mucus. In order to reach the fallopian tube and fertilize an egg therein, the sperm must first migrate through the cervical mucus. There are many factors that can impair the ability of the sperm to survive and traverse the cervical mucus, including faulty intercourse (*e.g,.* premature ejaculation), infection, prior surgery on the cervix and production of antibodies (substances that can kill or immobilize the sperm).

During a normal menstrual cycle, there are only a couple of days during which the sperm can survive in the cervical mucus. At other times of the cycle, the mucus is a very effective barrier. Around the time of ovulation, the cervical mucus becomes very thin and watery, and probably even somehow assists the sperm as they migrate through to the uterus and on to the fallopian tubes. The timing of this test is, therefore, crucial. If a woman's cycles are regular, an ovulation predictor test can be used. If she is on medication or has very irregular cycles, the timing of this test should be discussed with your physician, but must always be just prior to ovulation.

Have intercourse the morning of the post-coital test. Do not use lubricants or douche or take a bath after intercourse (showers are fine).

Note the approximate time of intercourse since that is important in evaluating the results. Although some authors state that this test must be done within two hours of intercourse, this is not important. Simply note how long it has been and notify your physician—they can adjust their interpretation based on the length of time.

In the office, a speculum exam is performed. A small amount of cervical mucus is withdrawn from the cervix (this is painless). This is then examined under the microscope. The quality of the cervical mucus as well as the number of sperm present and their motility will be assessed. You should be able to know the results right away.

If the post-coital test is abnormal, it should be repeated. This test is very dependent on proper timing in the cycle. If the test remains abnormal, there are a couple of possibilities:

1. Poor cervical mucus: Is there infection or prior surgery on the cervix, or is the woman on medications (*e.g.,* clomiphene) that might account for poor cervical mucus. Inseminations (see below) may be suggested as a means of dealing with this problem.

2. Poor sperm motility: This can suggest the presence of sperm antibodies. Sperm antibody testing should be considered. The presence of sperm antibodies would suggest that either inseminations or an ART procedure such as IVF or ZIFT be considered.

If the post-coital test is normal, evaluation of other possible factors should proceed. Sperm function testing should be considered before initiating treatments such as superovulation (Chapter 12), or an ART procedure.

Alternatives

If the semen analyses are repeatedly abnormal, sperm function testing and urologic referral should be obtained. If no significant improvement in the semen analysis is obtainable, then the TMNS should be calculated, the results of the sperm function testing taken into account, and the appropriate interventions or treatments considered. The number of TMNS that is adequate for each intervention will vary from lab to lab and physician to physician, but the alternatives include the following:

1. Inseminations (also known as AIH): A semen sample is collected (preferably by masturbation although intercourse with a special condom is

an option) and provided to the laboratory in a sterile specimen container. The semen sample obviously contains much more than just the sperm, including proteins, sugars and prostaglandins. The laboratory will treat the semen sample in such a fashion that a pure sperm sample suspended in a specially designed buffer is obtained. This sample is then placed in a small syringe to which is attached a small plastic tube, or catheter. A speculum is placed in the vagina, the catheter is directed through the cervix and into the uterus, and the sperm preparation is slowly injected. While this procedure may cause slight cramping, it is generally painless. This procedure allows a far greater number of sperm to reach the uterine cavity and fallopian tubes than would normally occur with intercourse.

2. ART (assisted reproductive technologies): These procedures will be discussed in detail in Chapter 13, but far fewer sperm are needed for these procedures to be successful than is the case even with inseminations, let alone intercourse.

3. ICSI (intracytoplasmic sperm injection): This too will be discussed in more detail in Chapter 13, but in short this procedure involves injecting a single sperm into an egg using a microscope and micromanipulation instruments. Fertilization and pregnancies can be achieved even if only a few sperm are present.

4. Donor sperm (Chapter 14): If there is complete absence of sperm (azoospermia), this may be the only option for achieving conception. Some couples will also opt to use donor sperm rather than resorting to some of the more high-tech procedures, often because of cost considerations.

Chapter Eight
The Female and The Fallopian Tubes

Overview: Tuboperitoneal Evaluation

Tuboperitoneal evaluation means making sure all of the pelvic structures, including the fallopian tubes, are in the right place, in proper relationship to one another, and capable of functioning. A couple of points about normal function must be kept in mind. When an egg is ovulated by the ovary, it doesn't just "pop" into the fallopian tube. The fimbria, or finger-like projections on the end of the tube near the ovary, must actively go and get the egg and "feed" it into the fallopian tube. The fimbria must, therefore, be in close proximity to the ovary. Secondly, the fallopian tube is not just some hollow tube that lets the egg fall into the uterus. It is a marvelously complex structure that nourishes the egg and early embryo, allows fertilization to occur, and actively transports the egg to meet the sperm and then transports the embryo into the uterus.

Causes of Tubal Problems

This evaluation obviously begins with a history and physical exam. There are several historical factors that may suggest a problem. As part of the initial evaluation, a pelvic exam should also be performed. The physician is trying to feel anything that would suggest a problem. Finally, a pelvic ultrasound is worthwhile on the initial visit. It allows the physician to look at the ovaries and be sure there are no cysts or other visible problems that might make surgery or other evaluation necessary. The combination of a good pelvic exam and an ultrasound will assure the physician that there is not significant endometriosis, which would dictate that laparoscopy is indicated.

Scar Tissue

Any prior pelvic surgery may result in adhesions, or scar tissue. Any time surgery is done, there is a chance that adhesions will form as a result of that surgery. And adhesions form very quickly: Following a surgery, most (if not all) of the adhesions that will form have done so within the first couple of weeks. Adhesions can significantly distort the normal relationship of the tubes and ovaries and can make it physically impossible for the fimbria to pick up the egg. Therefore, any prior history of pelvic surgery must be considered a possible predisposing factor for pelvic adhesions.

Infections

Infection is the leading cause of pelvic adhesions and damage to the fallopian tubes. Gonorrhea and chlamydia are the sexually transmitted organisms responsible for the vast majority of cases of salpingitis (inflammation of the fallopian tubes, also known as pelvic inflammatory disease or PID). Infection with gonorrhea is a very serious disease leading to high fever, pain, and other symptoms that alert one to its presence. Chlamydia, on the other hand, can infect and damage the fallopian tubes without causing any symptoms. *Chlamydia is the most common cause of tubal infection and damage, and a woman may never know she has had it.*
When a fallopian tube becomes infected, several things occur. One of the first changes to take place is damage to the cells that line the inside of the tube. Certain of these cells have what are known as "microcilia" on their surface. These microcilia are responsible for propelling the egg and embryo down the tube. When infection occurs, these microcilia are often damaged or destroyed, and they will not heal or reform. Secondly, it is a natural response of the body to try to contain an infection and prevent it from spreading. In attempting to do this, the fimbria of the tube close on each other. When scarring occurs, the fimbria may stay like this, thus closing off the tube and forming what is known as distal tubal disease. In severe cases, fluid may collect in the tube and form a hydrosalpinx, a dilated fallopian tube full of fluid. In other cases, there may be scarring and destruction of the part of the tube closest to the uterus, resulting in a change known as salpingitis isthmica nodosa (SIN).

Other sources of inflammation may also lead to tubal damage. Appendicitis, particularly if the appendix ruptured, can cause significant adhesions and tubal damage.

Endometriosis must also be considered as a potential cause of tuboperitoneal problems, but endometriosis is addressed separately in Chapter 9.

Methods of Evaluating Tubal Problems

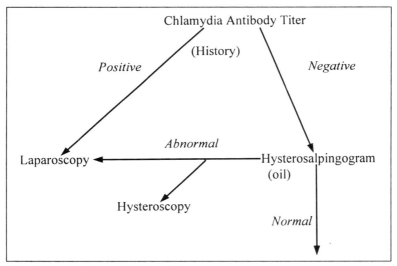

The Tuboperitoneal Algorithm

Chlamydia Antibody Titer

The tuboperitoneal algorithm is depicted in the chart. Virtually every patient experiencing difficulty conceiving should have what is known as a chlamydia antibody titer. This is a blood test that can detect whether or not a woman has ever been exposed to chlamydia. Since this infection can occur without any symptoms whatsoever, this blood test may provide the only evidence, short of surgical evaluation, that there has been an infection. The blood test provides no information about when the infection occurred; it simply tells us that there has been an infection at some point. Chlamydia may also infect areas other than the fallopian tubes, so a positive result does not necessarily mean that there has been a tubal infection. It is, however, suggestive enough that evaluation by laparoscopy is warranted.

If the chlamydia titer is negative (*i.e.*, there is no evidence of prior infection), if there is no history of prior surgery, and if no abnormalities are noted on the initial exam and ultrasound, the next step should be a hysterosalpingogram, not a laparoscopy.

Hysterosalpingogram

A hysterosalpingogram (HSG) is an X-ray procedure in which an iodine-based dye is injected through the cervix, into the uterus, and out through the fallopian tubes. This procedure is performed soon after a period ends but before ovulation occurs, usually between days seven and ten of the menstrual cycle. It is appropriate to give a two- or three-day course of antibiotics for this procedure since dye is being injected through the cervix and into the fallopian tubes. This reduces the risk of infection as a consequence of doing this procedure to less than one percent.

In the X-ray department, a speculum is placed in the vagina and a small instrument is attached to the cervix. Under fluoroscopy, which allows the physician to observe the procedure as it is being performed, dye is *slowly* injected and is observed as it first fills the uterine cavity, then proceeds into the fallopian tubes, and finally out the ends of the fallopian tubes into the abdominal cavity. X-rays are taken at key points during the procedure, and the entire procedure usually takes less than ten minutes. There may be some mild cramping after this procedure, but patients can usually return to work that same day without difficulty.

Usefulness of HSGs

HSGs are an excellent means of evaluating the uterine cavity to be sure that there is no scarring in the cavity, no polyps or other masses such as fibroids, which can distort the uterine cavity, and no uterine anomaly or abnormal shape. HSGs are also excellent for evaluating the internal appearance of the fallopian tube including the proximal segment, or isthmus, and for demonstrating that the tubes are open. In addition, there are a couple of important points to know about HSGs:

1. This does not have to be a terribly painful experience. Much of the pain often reported with HSGs occurs as a result of using instruments, such as balloons, that are placed into the uterine cavity. This can cause extreme cramping and discomfort. This procedure can be done every bit as well, if not better, by using instruments that are inserted only a short way into the cervix. This eliminates and avoids most of the discomfort. Mild to moderate menstrual cramping is the most that is usually experienced. Taking ibuprofen or some other mild pain reliever prior to the procedure will reduce the discomfort even further.

2. There is very good evidence that HSGs can be therapeutic as well as diagnostic. Conception rates improve for several months after an HSG (partly due, perhaps, to a simple flushing effect on the tubes, but also due to other effects of the X-ray contrast material). *However, this improvement of pregnancy rates after an HSG has been demonstrated only if the procedure is performed using oil-soluble contrast material.* I prefer to do the diagnostic part of the procedure using water-soluble contrast material, and then, having been assured that everything looks normal, inject the oil-soluble contrast material to obtain the therapeutic benefit.

(**Note:** HSGs are not the best procedure for evaluating the presence of scarring around the fallopian tubes or ovaries. While the physician may get some idea by observing the pattern of the spill of the dye from the tubes into the abdominal cavity [and this is one reason that the physician should observe the procedure under fluoroscopy while it is being done], the reliability of the HSG for evaluating for adhesions around the tube is not great. However, in the absence of prior infection or prior surgery and with no evidence of endometriosis, the chances of adhesions around the tubes should be very small indeed and the HSG is a very reliable and worthwhile procedure.)

If the HSG is normal, evaluation and treatment should continue with the assumption that the tuboperitoneal factor is normal. **There is no need to do a laparoscopy.** (Although mild or moderate endometriosis may still be present, this approach is valid. The rationale behind this is discussed fully in Chapter 9.)

Proximal Tubal Disease

If the HSG is abnormal, further evaluation is warranted. If the uterine cavity is abnormal, a hysteroscopy should be performed to further evaluate the abnormality and treat it. (Hysteroscopy is fully discussed in Chapter 10.) If the tubes are abnormal, unless the abnormality is proximal tubal disease, a laparoscopy should be considered to further evaluate and treat the abnormality. However, if severe tubal disease is present on the HSG, laparoscopy may not be warranted to surgically correct the tubes. IVF (in vitro fertilization) will offer much better pregnancy rates than will surgical correction. There is actually evidence to suggest that severely damaged tubes should be removed rather than corrected, in that IVF success rates appear to be higher if the tubes are removed (see Laparoscopy below).

There are several possible causes of proximal tubal disease or abnormalities of the portion of the tube immediately adjacent to the uterus:

Salpingitis isthmica nodosa (SIN)
> This is a destructive change related to an inflammatory process. This is best treated by proceeding to IVF. The other alternative is a major operative procedure in which the diseased portion of tube is removed and the remaining healthy tube is reconnected. This procedure carries a fifty percent chance of success at best, and IVF is probably a better alternative.

Proximal tubal occlusion
> HSGs will at times reveal proximal tubal occlusion because of mucus plugs, related to endometriosis, or for reasons that are unclear. Selective tubal cannulization (placing a small plastic catheter directly into the affected tube) can be performed at the time of the HSG. This will often result in clearing of this type of obstruction.

Tubal spasm
> On rare occasions, the tubes will go into spasm (like a muscle cramp) and will not allow the passage of dye. Using instruments that cause a minimum of uterine irritation will minimize the chances of this.

Laparoscopy

If the history is suggestive (*i.e.*, prior surgical procedures), if the chlamydia titer is positive (suggestive of prior infection), if the initial exam and ultrasound suggest significant endometriosis, or if the HSG is abnormal, laparoscopy should be the next step.

Laparoscopy is a minor surgical procedure that is performed under general anesthesia on an outpatient basis. A small instrument resembling a telescope and measuring less than half an inch in diameter is inserted just under the belly button. A small amount of gas is then introduced into the abdominal cavity, allowing complete visualization of the pelvic and abdominal organs. Often this procedure is videotaped to allow the patient to view the findings and procedure at a later date. Recovery in the hospital usually takes an hour or two. After a few days (at most) at home, recovery is usually complete and normal activity may be resumed.

Uses of Laparoscopy

Laparoscopy is a time-honored means of evaluating the ovaries, tubes and surrounding structures to see if they are normal, and laparoscopy certainly still has its place. It is one of the most valuable tools available to the physician evaluating and treating the subfertile female. But there are extremely rare circumstances under which it should be done simply for diagnostic purposes in evaluating infertility. *If a laparoscopy is done, it can be done as a potentially therapeutic procedure by which the physician can treat and correct virtually any pathology or abnormality found.*

One to three, or even four, additional small (5mm) incisions can be made in inconspicuous areas to allow the physician to introduce additional instruments for the purpose of operating and correcting abnormalities. The following surgical procedures can be done by laparoscopy: removal of adhesions, repair of the fallopian tubes, removal of ovarian cysts, treatment of endometriosis (laser, cautery, etc.), removal of ectopic pregnancies, removal of ovaries and/or tubes, appendectomy and hysterectomy.

The key point about laparoscopy is this—in the hands of an experienced laparoscopic surgeon, virtually any procedure that can be performed by a major surgical procedure (one performed through a major abdominal incision, and requiring a hospital stay and six to eight weeks of recovery) can be accomplished via laparoscopy. And there are significant advantages to a laparoscopic approach: Recovery is quicker and easier, and the results are as good if not better than those obtained by major surgery.

There's also this consideration. Let's suppose we do a laparoscopy and see that there are adhesions and distal tubal occlusion (the end of the tube by the ovary is blocked), perhaps as a result of a chlamydia infection. There are two options. We can go ahead and remove the adhesions and open the tubes at the time of the laparoscopy or we can see the problem, quit, and come back and do a major surgical procedure to remove the adhesions and open the tubes. In terms of chances of success, the two approaches are essentially equal in the hands of a skilled laparoscopic surgeon. In terms of patient suffering, inconvenience and disability, there is no comparison. In terms of financial liability, there is no question which approach makes better sense. *Be sure that you find out what the surgeon performing your laparoscopy intends to accomplish at the time of your laparoscopy.*

Evaluating Degrees of Tubal Damage and Assessing Treatments

There are certainly different degrees of tubal damage. It can range from a few thin and easily removed adhesions around the tube and ovary, to virtually complete destruction of the fallopian tube and very extensive adhesions. The chances of a successful pregnancy following surgical correction are directly related to the extent of the damage. Minimal disease can be corrected with up to a sixty percent or higher chance of successful pregnancy. Tubes that are severely damaged, on the other hand, may have only a three to five percent chance of working properly following surgery, whether it is major surgery or surgery performed laparoscopically. Again, there is good evidence that severely damaged tubes should be removed rather than corrected—correction results in very poor chances of successful pregnancy while removal seems to improve the success rate of IVF, which will be the more successful alternative anyway.

There are very few reasons to have major surgery for purposes of improving fertility. Removal of large fibroids and tubal reanastamosis following a tubal ligation (see below) are probably still best done via a major surgical approach. Virtually every other problem is best treated through the laparoscope. The chances of successful pregnancy following major surgery for treatment of severe tubal disease do not justify the pain and cost of the procedure. IVF is a better alternative: It costs less, is more successful, and is less invasive.

Tubal Ligation

One special category of tuboperitoneal factor is tubal occlusion as a result of a prior tubal ligation. There are many different reasons that individuals decide to try to have their tubes "untied," including remarriage and a simple desire for more children. The fallopian tubes are, however, never actually "tied." There are many different ways of doing a tubal ligation, but they all involve destroying at least a small portion of the tube. This can range from removal of a small piece of the tube to destruction or removal of the entire tube. Some tubal ligations can be reversed (the tubes put back together), and some can't. In general, the more of the tube that was destroyed at the time of the tubal ligation, the poorer the chances of successful function after tubal reanastamosis are. The use of cautery to do a tubal ligation also makes it less likely that the tubes can be repaired. If, however, only a small piece of tube is missing, surgery for putting the tubes back together (reanastamosis) is very successful, with postsurgery pregnancy rates as high as eighty percent.

Office Laparoscopy

There has been some interest generated lately in a procedure known as *office laparoscopy*. This involves the use of very small instruments (2 mm), and the procedure is done under local anesthesia in an office-type setting. The advantages of this procedure are the cost savings associated with doing the procedure in the office rather than in an operating room, and the fact that it is done under local rather than general anesthesia. However, there are some significant limitations to this procedure. In fact, at the current time, this is essentially a purely diagnostic procedure, although some simple and quick procedures such as tubal ligation or gamete intrafallopian transfer (GIFT) can be done very effectively using this technique. And office laparoscopy may have some role in helping a physician determine the cause of a woman's pelvic pain.

But office laparoscopy currently does not have much of a role in evaluating the infertile woman. We have already seen that unless there is a significant index of suspicion of tubal disease, HSG is the preferred method of tubal evaluation. HSGs are still much less invasive and much less expensive than office laparoscopy. And we also know that if we are going to do a laparoscopy, we might as well be prepared to correct whatever pathology we encounter. Office laparoscopy does not allow one to do longer, more involved surgeries such as repairing fallopian tubes, removing adhesions or lasering endometriosis. If significant pathology is encountered, another surgical procedure must be scheduled at a later date to correct that problem. Doing an office laparoscopy would, in essence, be the same as doing a laparoscopy and then coming back and doing a major surgery at a later date. *If there is enough of a reason to do a surgical procedure, it makes more sense to do one that allows correction of a problem, not one that may result in yet another surgery.*

Saline Infusion Sonohysterography

Saline infusion sonohysterography is a relatively new technique. It allows one to assess the uterine cavity, and to a certain extent, the fallopian tubes in the office using ultrasound. At the time of a pelvic exam, a small catheter is placed through the cervix and into the uterus. The speculum is removed and the vaginal ultrasound probe is introduced. Saline is slowly injected through the catheter and the outlines of the uterine cavity are evaluated. This is an excellent means of evaluating the uterine cavity for abnormalities such as polyps, fibroids and congenital anomalies. Its utility, however, is somewhat limited by the compromised evaluation and visualization of the fallopian tubes, which it provides. It does not allow nearly the accuracy or detail that an HSG does in terms of the status of the tubes. As we have discussed above, we rely fairly heavily on the results of the HSG. The HSG may very well be the only form of tubal evaluation we perform. I do not feel that the reliability and accuracy of saline infusion sonohysterograpy are good enough to use it instead of the HSG for tubal evaluation. Furthermore, there is no evidence that doing saline infusion sonohysterography improves conception rates following the procedure. Therefore, I much prefer HSG for tubal evaluation. If we are simply interested in evaluating the uterine cavity for abnormalities; saline infusion sonohysterography is a perfectly appropriate means of doing so.

CHAPTER NINE
THE FEMALE AND ENDOMETRIOSIS

OVERVIEW: ENDOMETRIOSIS

Every month when a woman has a period, the cells that line the uterus, known as the endometrium, are shed in the menstrual flow. Some small portion of this combination of blood and endometrial cells may also pass out through the fallopian tubes into the abdominal cavity. Most of the time, the body's natural defense systems attack and destroy these cells before they can begin to grow. However, for reasons that are not clear, this is not always the case. In certain individuals, these endometrial cells actually implant on structures in the abdominal cavity and begin to grow. *This is endometriosis: the presence of viable endometrial cells in places other than the uterine cavity.* Then, each month when the normal hormonal changes result in a menstrual period, much the same change occurs in the endometriosis. A small amount of bleeding occurs from the endometriosis cells. This is very irritating to the body, and as a result of this, scarring occurs around the endometriosis. Most often this is a progressive process, with a small additional amount of bleeding and scarring occurring every month.

Once the endometrial cells begin to grow in the abdominal cavity, they are known as implants. Implants can occur on any structure, including the ovaries, fallopian tubes, bladder, bowel and on the lining of the abdominal cavity (known as the *peritoneum*). The area behind the uterus, between it and the rectum, is known as the cul-de-sac, and this is the most common site for endometriosis. Implants may appear as small, clear or red, fluid-filled sacs, or most commonly, as dark brown or black areas. It is the collection of old blood in the implants that gives them this appearance. Some scarring is typical around the implants, and can be very localized or, at times, quite severe. When endometriosis develops in the ovaries, large cysts full of old blood, known as *chocolate cysts* or *endometriomas*, may result.

There are other theories as to how endometriosis develops, and this scenario (known as *retrograde menstruation*) certainly cannot explain all cases of endometriosis. It is, however, the most widely held theory and does explain all but the most unusual cases of endometriosis.

Although in some individuals endometriosis may cause no symptoms, it is typically associated with two problems: difficulty conceiving and pain. The pain may be present as extremely painful menstrual periods. In the presence of endometriosis, the pain with the periods, known as *dysmenorrhea*, often becomes worse as one gets older. Pain with intercourse is not uncommon in women with endometriosis, and there may even be pain that persists throughout the month but is worse during periods. Not everyone with endometriosis has pain; in fact, there is little correlation between the amount of endometriosis an individual has and the amount of pain she experiences. Sometimes a single, small implant may cause excruciating pain, while someone with severe disease may be pain free.

The association of endometriosis with difficulty conceiving has long been known, and research has demonstrated many different ways in which endometriosis interferes with normal conception. Endometrial implants are irritating to the body, and as a result of this, the body produces a group of substances known as *prostaglandins*. Prostaglandins have been shown to alter not only the maturation and development of the egg within the ovary, but also the release of the egg from the ovary. The ability of the tube to function normally may also be impaired. Whereas in "nature's way" the tube is poised and ready to pick up an egg if one appears on the surface of the ovary, in the presence of endometriosis the tube may be "lazy" or "floppy." Not only is the overall tone of the tube decreased, but the fimbria, which are responsible for egg pickup, may end up being very far from the ovary itself. The combination of these factors may make it very difficult for the tube to pick the egg up off the surface of the ovary. Thus, even if ovulation does occur, the egg may not get into the fallopian tube. Endometrial implants also result in the increased production and increased activation of a group of cells known as *macrophages*. Macrophages are part of the body's natural defense system and can be visualized as little "Pac-men," actively attacking and destroying any cells that they encounter. One of the groups of cells that macrophages attack and destroy more than normal in women with endometriosis are the sperm, thus making it more difficult for the sperm to reach and fertilize the egg. The macrophages may also interfere with tubal function, ovarian function, and perhaps even early embryo development. It is important to keep in mind the number and variety of ways endometriosis affects fertility, particularly when discussing the ways of treating endometriosis.

DIAGNOSING ENDOMETRIOSIS

It is not clear why endometriosis occurs in some individuals and not in others, but about ten to twenty percent of all reproductive-age females have been found to have endometriosis. In women with infertility, this number may be as high as thirty to fifty percent. Factors associated with the development of endometriosis include delayed childbearing, long periods of uninterrupted menstrual cycles, abnormal pelvic anatomy and stress. Many other factors have been associated with the development of endometriosis and there is even a genetic factor, meaning that one may inherit an increased likelihood of developing this process if a close relative has it.

The physician can often suspect endometriosis on the basis of a history and physical exam. A history of progressively worsening pain with the menstrual periods is suggestive. A history of cramping that begins two to three days before the onset of menstrual bleeding is also common with endometriosis, as is deep dyspareunia (pain with deep penetration at the time of intercourse). During the physical exam, the physician may be able to feel endometriosis, particularly if it is in the cul-de-sac. Endometriosis is not visible by ultrasound unless there is ovarian involvement; endometriomas are visible by ultrasound. If significant endometriosis is present, the combination of a history, pelvic exam and ultrasound will reveal it.

There are tremendous variations in the amount of endometriosis an individual may have. The American Society for Reproductive Medicine has developed a grading system for quantifying the amount of endometriosis present (see chart). While there are many limitations to this system of classification, it does provide a means for comparing the extent of endometriosis from patient to patient and may be useful in prognosticating about the chances of conceiving. The only way to definitively diagnose endometriosis is by visualizing the process at the time of surgery. At the time of laparoscopy, the surgeon notes the endometriosis present and any adhesions or scarring that may have formed as a result of the endometriosis. These findings are then recorded on the classification sheet and a score assigned. That score is then used to determine the grade of disease, ranging from mild to extensive. (See forms at end of chapter.)

MEDICAL THERAPIES

Before discussing any form of medical therapy, it is important to stress that *there is no medical therapy that cures endometriosis. All forms of medical therapy must be seen as means of temporarily suppressing the process only, not as ways of curing it.*

Endometrial implants are dependent on cyclic hormonal function, such as occurs in a normal menstrual cycle. All forms of medical therapy are aimed at disrupting cyclic hormone production and creating a state in which the hormones are constant from day to day. When estrogen and progesterone are steady from day to day over a prolonged period of time, endometriosis typically does not progress, and may even regress. There are two normal physiological states in a woman's life during which her hormones are essentially constant from day to day—pregnancy and menopause. Medical therapies aim to simulate one of these states.

Pseudopregnancy

In the majority of women, endometriosis improves during pregnancy. During pregnancy, ovulation stops and relatively constant, high levels of estrogen and progesterone are present. One can simulate these high constant levels of hormones, or create a state of "pseudopregnancy," by the use of birth control pills. The birth control pills suppress ovulation and result in a steady state of relatively high hormone levels, just as is seen in pregnancy. To effect this pseudopregnancy, the pill must be taken continuously. In other words, a pill is taken every day without ever stopping for a week or without taking the "sugar pills" at the end of the pack. Thus, no periods will occur because a hormonally active pill is being taken every day, and a steady hormone state is achieved. For women who can take the pill, this is a perfectly safe way to do so. Because of the balance of the hormones in the pill, the lining of the uterus does not build up while on continuous therapy, and if anything, it actually thins out. There is no need to have a period each month while on the pill. If the pill is being used to treat or suppress endometriosis, having a period each month will probably render the pill far less effective because of the bleeding and resulting changes in the endometrial implants.

Pseudomenopause

Suppressing Ovary Function

There are basically two types of medications available for creating a state of pseudomenopause. The first of these is danocrine (Danazol). This is an attenuated, or altered, male hormone. When taken in adequate doses, it results in suppression of the ovaries such that they temporarily stop functioning. This combination of decreased female hormone levels and increased male hormone levels accounts for much of the effectiveness of danocrine in suppressing endometriosis. Danocrine has been around for years and for a long time was the most commonly used form of medical suppression. It does, however, have many unpleasant side effects, including menopausal symptoms such as hot flashes and vaginal dryness. In addition, side effects related to the fact that it is a derivative of a male hormone, such as weight gain, increased muscle mass, hirsutism (increased hair growth) and muscle cramps limit the acceptability of danocrine. With the availability of the GnRH agonists, danocrine is not widely used to treat endometriosis at this time.

Suppressing Pituitary Production

The GnRH agonists are a class of medications that can temporarily suppress the ability of the pituitary to produce LH and FSH. If the pituitary does not produce LH and FSH, the ovaries receive no stimulation and therefore stop producing hormones. Thus, once again, a temporary state of menopause is achieved. The most commonly used form of this therapy is the depo, or long-acting, form of leuprolide acetate, known as Depo-Lupron. An injection of this medication given once a month results in very effective suppression of the ovaries. The major side effects associated with this medication are menopause-related ones, specifically hot flashes and vaginal dryness. In some individuals, these side effects may be severe. Although it may somewhat limit the overall effectiveness of the therapy, small doses of estrogen may be administered along with the Depo-Lupron. A minimal dose of estrogen makes this therapy very tolerable for most individuals. If a small enough dose of estrogen is used, often the side effects can be eliminated without significantly compromising the effectiveness of the treatment.

Precautions in Using Suppressive Therapies

While on suppressive therapies, particularly those that induce pseudomenopause, it is important to take a good multivitamin as well as some calcium supplementation. The lack of estrogen does result in the potential for development of at least a small amount of osteoporosis, or thinning of the bones, while on this therapy. The calcium and vitamins help to minimize this potential sideeffect. However, because of the potential development of osteoporosis and other menopause-related side effects, the length of time that these therapies may be used is limited. Although circumstances may dictate special considerations for some individuals, six months of therapy is usually considered maximal.

All forms of suppressive therapy must be viewed as exactly that—a means of suppressing the endometriosis. The endometriosis will not, in the vast majority of cases, progress while on this therapy. In most cases it actually improves. *Suppressive therapies do not, however, cure the endometriosis.* Upon their discontinuation, normal menstrual function resumes and the endometrial implants, which had been suppressed, also begin to function and respond to the cyclic hormone changes. Often within a relatively brief period of time, the endometriosis is right back where it was before the treatment was begun. Suppressive therapies should be viewed only as ways of buying time. If you know you have endometriosis and want to get pregnant, but for one reason or another must postpone your attempts to do so for another six months, then suppressive therapy may be a great idea. *Suppressive therapy does not improve one's chances of getting pregnant.* There is no data to suggest that medical therapy results in improved chances of conceiving. This is also true regarding its use after surgery for endometriosis. Suppressive therapy after surgery for endometriosis does little if anything to improve one's chances of getting pregnant. It is a good way to buy some time during which the endometriosis will not get worse; it is not a good way to improve your chances of getting pregnant.

SURGICAL TREATMENTS

The obvious goal of surgical therapy is the elimination of all the endometrial implants. There are many different techniques for surgically treating endometriosis, but there are two important principles that need to be stressed right from the beginning and that will be explained in more detail later: *1) rarely is a major surgical procedure indicated to treat endometriosis for purposes of increasing your chances of getting pregnant, and 2) if there is no alteration of normal anatomy as a result of scarring from endometriosis, surgery to eliminate the endometriosis does not improve one's chances of getting pregnant.*

For Treatment of Scarring and Associated Pain

Surgical therapy for endometriosis must be considered from the standpoint of the two major symptoms of endometriosis; that is, pain and infertility. Let's first deal with pain. As noted above, endometrial implants are small collections of blood surrounded by scarring. The progressive nature of these implants causes more blood to accumulate while the scarring around it increases, often causing severe pain. The surgical eradication of these implants is an excellent means of improving if not eliminating endometriosis-associated pain. Again, even a small single implant can cause severe pain and there is little correlation between the amount of endometriosis present and the amount of pain. Therefore, if the history and physical exam are suggestive enough, laparoscopy and destruction of any endometriosis encountered should be considered for the potential relief of pain.

Laparoscopy

Laparoscopy is a minor surgical procedure done under general anesthesia and usually performed on an outpatient basis. A small incision less than an inch long is made under the belly button and a telescopelike instrument is inserted. A small amount of carbon dioxide is placed in the abdominal cavity to allow the surgeon to see the abdominal and pelvic organs. One to three additional incisions less than a quarter inch may also be used to introduce additional instruments. Through the laparoscope, the surgeon should be able to treat all but the most severe cases of endometriosis. Full recovery usually takes only a few days. Major surgery is typically required only if there is significant involvement of the bowel with endometriosis.

Lasers

The means by which the endometrial implants are destroyed seems to be inconsequential. There are several different types of lasers available, including carbon dioxide, argon, KTP and YAG. One can also use electro-cautery. It doesn't matter! All that is important is that the cells of the implant are destroyed without causing significant damage to the surrounding tissue. Surgical therapy for pain associated with endometriosis is often a very effective procedure and can result in a tremendous decrease in the amount of pain an individual experiences.

For Treatment of Infertility

Surgical therapy for endometriosis-associated infertility is an entirely different matter. *If there is no significant alteration of normal pelvic anatomy as a result of scarring associated with endometriosis, there is little if any improvement of conception rates as a result of surgical treatment of the endometriosis.* If one has less than moderate endometriosis according the classification depicted above, there is no benefit to doing a laparoscopy and destroying the lesions. How does one know how much endometriosis there is unless one does a laparoscopy to find out? First of all, the physician has done a pelvic exam, which will provide reliable information about pelvic anatomy. Secondly, the initial pelvic ultrasound has revealed whether or not there is an endometrioma present in the ovaries. It is very uncommon to have moderate endometriosis without some ovarian involvement that will be visible on ultrasound, or significant findings on the pelvic exam. Therefore, a good initial evaluation will allow a reliable determination of the potential extent of disease.

If there is ovarian involvement or significant scarring (adhesions) present, laparoscopic surgical intervention is warranted. Any endometrioma(s) can be removed from the ovaries, any adhesions cut and removed and all visible lesions destroyed. This can and should all be done through the laparoscope rather than with major surgery. Aside from the fact that recovery is much easier and quicker for a laparoscopy than for major surgery, studies have shown that the results achieved from laparoscopic treatment are every bit as good if not better than those achieved with major surgery. The technology and instrumentation necessary to perform thorough treatment for all but the most severe cases of endometriosis through the laparoscope are available. If you are going to have a laparoscopy to evaluate for the presence of endometriosis, ask your surgeon how she or he intends to treat it. Do not have major surgery to treat endometriosis unless it is determined to be very severe.

If the initial evaluation suggests that there is not moderate or severe endometriosis present, there is probably no need to have a laparoscopy. There is no rationale for doing a laparoscopy to treat minimal or mild disease when dealing with endometriosis-associated infertility. Many studies have been done. All but one of these studies demonstrate that surgical treatment of mild endometriosis is not associated with any improvement in the chances of getting pregnant. This makes sense! You will recall that there are many mechanisms by which endometriosis impairs fertility. None of these are really altered by eliminating the endometrial implants. For example, if the endometriosis has altered the motility or ability of the fallopian tube to pick up an egg from the ovary, it is difficult to imagine that treating the implants will restore this function. The same is true for most of the other proposed mechanisms of endometriosis-associated infertility. There is ample evidence showing that the chances of getting pregnant with mild endometriosis are the same whether one pursues "expectant management" (simple continued attempts at conceiving without any intervention) or has a laparoscopy to destroy the endometriosis. Couples with infertility associated with endometriosis without anatomic alteration should be treated and approached like couples with unexplained infertility, and this does not include doing a laparoscopy (Chapter 12).

Overall, the chances of successfully conceiving with endometriosis are inversely proportional to the extent of the disease: The worse the endometriosis is, the harder it becomes to get pregnant. Fortunately, truly severe endometriosis is uncommon. Exact percentages obviously are very individual, but with proper management and treatment, the vast majority of women with endometriosis will successfully conceive.

Finally, if you have mild endometriosis and are going to have a laparoscopy for purposes of helping you conceive, use that laparoscopy to do GIFT (Chapter 13). Pregnancy rates as high as forty to fifty percent can be achieved after a single laparoscopy and a GIFT procedure. This percentage is far better than that which can be achieved following a laparoscopy and laser or cautery of endometriosis. And GIFT works just as well if endometriosis is present as it does if the endometriosis has previously been treated.

All of this certainly does not imply that there are not circumstances under which surgery is the preferred form of therapy for endometriosis. Obviously, there will be cases and circumstances where surgical intervention for endometriosis is clearly indicated. But the point is this: In the past, the possibility of finding a small amount of endometriosis and treating it has been the justification for many, many surgical procedures. Some individuals have actually had several laparoscopies, or even major surgeries, for this reason. Not only is this invasive, in that an individual must endure one or more surgical procedures, it is also expensive. There are far more effective ways of achieving pregnancy—ones that are more cost-effective and far less invasive. Some of these approaches will be discussed in the chapter on unexplained infertility, and alternative treatments available are detailed in the chapter on ovulation induction (particularly gonadotropins) and in the chapter on the ART procedures.

THE AMERICAN FERTILITY SOCIETY
REVISED CLASSIFICATION OF ENDOMETRIOSIS

Patient's Name _____ Date_____

Stage I   (Minimal) - 1-5
Stage II (Mild)   - 6-15
Stage III (Moderate) - 16-40
Stage IV (Severe)   - >40
Total_____

Laparoscopy_____ Laparotomy_____ Photography_____
Recommended Treatment_____
_____
Prognosis_____

PERITONEUM	**ENDOMETRIOSIS**	<1cm	1-3cm	>3cm
	Superficial	1	2	4
	Deep	2	4	6
OVARY	R Superficial	1	2	4
	Deep	4	16	20
	L Superficial	1	2	4
	Deep	4	16	20

	POSTERIOR CULDESAC OBLITERATION	Partial	Complete
		4	40

	ADHESIONS	<1/3 Enclosure	1/3-2/3 Enclosure	>2/3 Enclosure
OVARY	R Filmy	1	2	4
	Dense	4	8	16
	L Filmy	1	2	4
	Dense	4	8	16
TUBE	R Filmy	1	2	4
	Dense	4*	8*	16
	L Filmy	1	2	4
	Dense	4*	8*	16

*If the fimbriated end of the fallopian tube is completely enclosed, change the point assignment to 16.

Additional Endometriosis: _____
_____
_____
_____

Associated Pathology: _____
_____
_____
_____

To Be Used with Normal
Tubes and Ovaries

L   R

To Be Used with Abnormal
Tubes and/or Ovaries

L   R

Reprinted by permission from the American Society for Reproductive Medicine
(*Fertility and Sterility*, Vol 67, No. 5, pp 819-820)

STAGE I (MINIMAL) STAGE II (MILD) STAGE III (MODERATE)

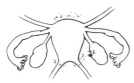

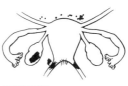

PERITONEUM
Superficial Endo — 1-3cm - 2
R. OVARY
Superficial Endo — ⟨ 1cm - 1
Filmy Adhesions — ⟨ 1/3 - 1
TOTAL POINTS 4

PERITONEUM
Deep Endo — ⟩3cm - 6
R. OVARY
Superficial Endo — ⟨ 1cm - 1
Filmy Adhesions — ⟨ 1/3 - 1
L. OVARY
Superficial Endo — ⟨1cm - 1
TOTAL POINTS 9

PERITONEUM
Deep Endo — ⟩3cm - 6
CULDESAC
Partial Obliteration - 4
L. OVARY
Deep Endo — 1-3cm - 16
TOTAL POINTS 26

STAGE III (MODERATE) STAGE IV (SEVERE) STAGE IV (SEVERE)

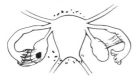

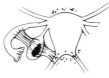

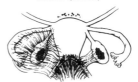

PERITONEUM
Superficial Endo — ⟩3cm -4
R. TUBE
Filmy Adhesions — ⟨ 1/3 - 1
R. OVARY
Filmy Adhesions — ⟨ 1/3 - 1
L. TUBE
Dense Adhesions — ⟨ 1/3 - 16*
L. OVARY
Deep Endo — ⟨1 cm -4
Dense Adhesions — ⟨ 1/3 -4
TOTAL POINTS 30

PERITONEUM
Superficial Endo — ⟩3cm -4
L. OVARY
Deep Endo — 1-3cm - 32**
Dense Adhesions — ⟨ 1/3 - 8**
L. TUBE
Dense Adhesions — ⟨ 1/3 -8**
TOTAL POINTS 52

*Point assignment changed to 16
**Point assignment doubled

PERITONEUM
Deep Endo — ⟩3cm - 6
CULDESAC
Complete Obliteration - 40
R. OVARY
Deep Endo — 1-3cm - 16
Dense Adhesions — ⟨ 1/3 - 4
L. TUBE
Dense Adhesions — ⟩2/3 - 16
L. OVARY
Deep Endo — 1-3cm - 16
Dense Adhesions — ⟩2/3 - 16
TOTAL POINTS 114

Determination of the stage or degree of endometrial involvement is based on a weighted point system. Distribution of points has been arbitrarily determined and may require further revision or refinement as knowledge of the disease increases.

To ensure complete evaluation, inspection of the pelvis in a clockwise or counterclockwise fashion is encouraged. Number, size and location of endometrial implants, plaques, endometriomas and/or adhesions are noted. For example, five separate 0.5cm superficial implants on the peritoneum (2.5 cm total) would be assigned 2 points. (The surface of the uterus should be considered peritoneum.) The severity of the endometriosis or adhesions should be assigned the highest score only for peritoneum, ovary, tube or culdesac. For example, a 4cm superficial and a 2cm deep implant of the peritoneum should be given a score of 6 (not 8). A 4cm

deep endometrioma of the ovary associated with more than 3cm of superficial disease should be scored 20 (not 24).

In those patients with only one adenexa, points applied to disease of the remaining tube and ovary should be multipled by two. ''Points assigned may be circled and totaled. Aggregation of points indicates stage of disease (minimal, mild, moderate, or severe).

The presence of endometriosis of the bowel, urinary tract, fallopian tube, vagina, cervix, skin etc., should be documented under "additional endometriosis." Other pathology such as tubal occlusion, leiomyomata, uterine anomaly, etc., should be documented under "associated pathology." All pathology should be depicted as specifically as possible on the sketch of pelvic organs, and means of observation (laparoscopy or laparotomy) should be noted.

Chapter Ten
The Female, the Cervix and the Uterus

Impaired fertility related to problems of the cervix and uterus is relatively rare, but certainly does occur, and evaluation of these factors must be included.

Overview: The Cervix

Cervical mucus is produced by a group of cells that line the inside of the cervix known as columnar cells. The cervical mucus is really quite remarkable. During the vast majority of the cycle, it is an extremely effective barrier that prevents anything from entering into the uterus. However, for a few days just prior to ovulation, it changes dramatically. As a result of stimulation by estrogen, which is produced by the cells surrounding the maturing egg, the cervical mucus becomes very clear, almost watery, and probably actually helps rather than hinders the sperm as they try to migrate through on their way to the fallopian tubes. As soon as ovulation occurs and progesterone production begins as a result thereof, the mucus again becomes thick and impenetrable.

Evaluation: The Postcoital Test

The best way to evaluate the cervical mucus is through the post-coital test, the performance and timing of which is discussed in detail in Chapter 4. In short, the post-coital test involves checking the interaction of the sperm and mucus by looking at the cervical mucus shortly after intercourse. The characteristics of the mucus which can be evaluated include:

Ferning. When the cervical mucus dries on a microscope slide, it should take on the appearance of ferns. This assures that the mucus has been exposed to adequate levels of estrogen without any exposure to progesterone; in other words, that the timing is correct.

Amount. Cervical mucus production normally increases dramatically just prior to ovulation.

Clarity. It should be very clear, almost watery.

Cellularity. There should be relatively few cells present, other than sperm.

Spinnbarkeit. This is the stretchiness of the cervical mucus. It should be almost elastic and may stretch ten centimeters or more.

Causes of Cervical Mucus Problems

There are several reasons why the cervical mucus may be poor and account for a bad post-coital test:

Poor Timing of the Test. This is far and away the most common reason that a post-coital test is unsatisfactory. This test must be performed just before ovulation occurs, when the cervical mucus is optimal.

Infection. The cells lining the cervix may become irritated or even infected. This will often be indicated by the presence of white blood cells in the mucus.

Prior Procedures on the Cervix. The cervical mucus is produced by the columnar cells that normally line the inside of the cervix. When these cells are damaged or destroyed, the normal repair process replaces them with a type of cell known as squamous cells. These squamous cells are incapable of making cervical mucus. Therefore, destruction of enough of the columnar cells can lead to a dramatic decrease in cervical mucus production. Procedures that can result in this type of change include freezing of the cervix, laser to the cervix, lleetz or leep procedures and cervical conizations, all of which are performed to treat abnormal Pap smears.

Medications. The most notable of these is clomiphene. Clomiphene can dramatically impair cervical mucus quantity and quality. Anyone on clomiphene, or anyone who has had her dose of clomiphene increased, should have a post-coital test checked. (Clomiphene is an antiestrogen. It literally blocks the effect of estrogen on cells. Estrogen induces the columnar cells in the cervix to produce mucus; clomiphene can block this effect.)

Treatment of Cervical Problems
Tetracyclines

The presence of white blood cells suggesting an infection can usually be resolved by treating the woman with an antibiotic. Tetracyclines are most commonly used for this purpose.

Cough Medicines

In certain individuals, there may be some role for cough medicines. Certain cough medicines (*e.g., Robitussin*) contain substances (*e.g.,* guaifenesin) that actually do help thin out the cervical mucus. Taking a teaspoon three or four times a day for the two or three days before ovulation may result in some thinning of the mucus.

Estrogen

If a woman is on a certain dose of clomiphene and seems to be ovulating well but the cervical mucus is poor, some physicians will prescribe small doses of estrogen. The thinking here is that giving some additional estrogen may override the blocking effect of the clomiphene and improve cervical mucus production. While this approach is safe and easy, if it does not result in significant improvement (as checked by the post-coital test), inseminations should be considered instead.

Inseminations

Inseminations are a means of bypassing the cervical mucus altogether. A semen sample is provided by masturbation and then prepared by the laboratory so that a pure preparation of sperm is suspended in a specially prepared salt buffer. This preparation is then placed in a small syringe that is attached to a small plastic catheter. A speculum is placed in the vagina and the catheter is gently guided through the cervix and into the uterus. This is a painless, nonsurgical procedure and is particularly useful if the mucus producing cells of the cervix are destroyed or nonfunctional. The cervical mucus is, in essence, bypassed by placing the sperm beyond the cervix and into the uterus.

OVERVIEW: THE UTERUS

The uterus is a remarkable organ. It is comprised primarily of muscle, known as *myometrium*. When nonpregnant, it is about the size and shape of a small pear, but during pregnancy it can expand to hold a full-term infant. After delivery, it can then contract back down to essentially its original size. The cervix is the part of the uterus that opens into the vagina, and the main part of the uterus is known as the fundus. The cavity of the uterus, which when not pregnant is very small, is lined by a group of cells called the *endometrium*. It is these cells that undergo the regular monthly changes as a result of the hormones produced by the ovaries. These changes either allow implantation and a pregnancy to occur, or result in a menstrual period. The diagram depicts in schematic fashion the changes that occur in the endometrium on a monthly basis. The first half of the menstrual cycle, the time from the start of the period until ovulation, is known as the *proliferative phase* because it is during this time that the lining of the uterus is thickening (proliferating). The part of the cycle between ovulation and the next period is known as the *secretory phase* because the lining is undergoing changes that will allow a pregnancy to implant should one occur. When a period occurs, this tissue is all shed and the whole cycle starts over again.

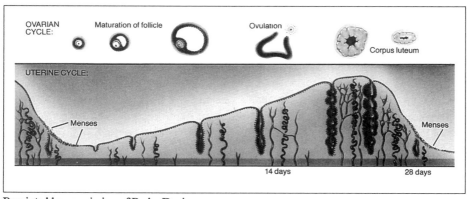

Reprinted by permission of Parke-Davis

ANATOMIC PROBLEMS OF THE UTERUS

All of the anatomic problems of the uterus can be detected by either a physical exam, a hysterosalpingogram (an X-ray procedure, which is discussed in Chapter 7), or by hysteroscopy (a surgical procedure in which a small instrument is inserted into the uterus and the uterine cavity visualized). If the hysterosalpingogram suggests that the uterine cavity is abnormal or the history and physical exam suggest such a problem may exist, hysteroscopy should be performed. Although diagnostic hysteroscopy can be performed in the office, any procedure done to correct an abnormality is probably best done in the operating room. Under anesthesia, a small instrument that is connected to a light source is inserted through the cervix and into the uterus. The uterine cavity is distended using one of a number of different agents that affords the surgeon a better view of the inside of the uterus. Small surgical instruments can be introduced through the hysteroscope including scissors, lasers and a variety of other instruments that allow the surgeon to correct many abnormalities. Polyps, fibroids, scarring of the uterine cavity and some uterine anomalies can all be corrected this way.

Anomalies

When the uterus is formed, it begins as two tubelike structures that begin on the side of the pelvis and come together in the middle. When they come together, the tissue in the middle is resorbed and the cavity is formed. In a small percentage of women, this process does not occur properly, and various anomalies can result. Some of these are depicted below. While few, if any, of these are associated with infertility, they may have other consequences such as recurrent pregnancy loss (see Chapter 15 for a full discussion).

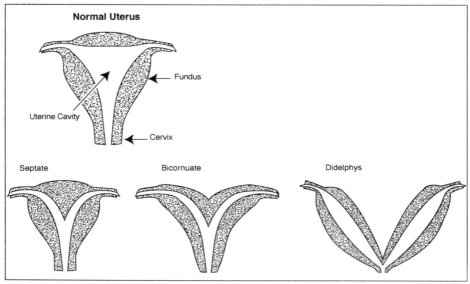

Some Types of Uterine Anomalies

Fibroids

Technically known as leiomyomas, these are benign (99+% of the time) muscle tumors that grow in the uterus. No one knows what causes fibroids, but there certainly is good evidence that there is a genetic predisposition. If your mother or sister has them, you are more likely to. Fibroids may be very small or extremely large, ranging in size from pea size to as big as a grapefruit or larger. Most fibroids do not cause difficulty conceiving. However, there are exceptions. A large fibroid that distorts pelvic anatomy so that the fallopian tubes cannot function properly can certainly be significant. Also, any fibroid that distorts the uterine cavity can be a problem.

If a fibroid distorts the uterine cavity enough that it can be seen on X-ray or by hysteroscopy, it has probably compromised the blood supply to the endometrium that overlies it. If this blood supply is compromised, this tissue cannot function properly and undergo all of the changes that it should, and it may not be able to allow implantation. Fibroids can also be pedunculated, or hanging into the uterine cavity from a stalk. The uterus does not like having anything in it with the exception of a fetus. Fibroids in the uterine cavity can result in much the same effect that occurs with an IUD—they irritate the uterus enough that it will not allow implantation to occur. Fibroids that distort the uterine cavity may be associated with bleeding at times other than the normal period. Consideration should be given to removing any fibroid within the uterine cavity or that distorts the uterine cavity.

Polyps

Polyps are overgrowths of the endometrium that almost resemble stalactites in a cave. They can result in effects much like an IUD, and may also be associated with abnormal bleeding.

Scarring

Sometimes after a D&C, particularly if it is done around the time of a pregnancy, scarring may occur. One wall of the uterus actually sticks to the other wall. This is known as intrauterine synechiae, or Asherman's syndrome. This scarring may be minimal, with one small band of scar tissue, or severe, at times almost obliterating the entire uterine cavity.

TREATMENT OF UTERINE PROBLEMS

Most of these problems can be adequately evaluated and treated with a hysteroscopy. There are many instruments, including scissors and lasers, that can be inserted through the hysteroscope and used to operate. Scarring and polyps can certainly be addressed in this fashion, as can pedunculated fibroids. Some smaller fibroids can also be removed in this fashion, but at times larger ones require major abdominal surgery for removal.

Uterine septums, as depicted above, can be removed quite adequately by hysteroscopy, often times by just incising them with scissors.

Some of the other anomalies, such as a bicornuate uterus, require major surgery for reconstruction.

FUNCTIONAL UTERINE PROBLEMS

Knowledge in much of this area is being gained rapidly, but is relatively new. There are a few problems that can be discussed.

Luteal Phase Defect

This is a defect in which the endometrium either is not exposed to enough progesterone or does not respond properly to the progesterone that is produced. As a result, the cells of the endometrium do not undergo the very orderly series of changes that they must undergo to allow implantation to occur. Consequently, even if a conception does occur, the endometrium may not be ready to accept it and, therefore, implantation will not occur. In the past, this has been diagnosed by an endometrial biopsy, an invasive and sometimes painful procedure in which a small piece of the lining of the uterus is removed and analyzed for proper development under the microscope.

You do not necessarily need to have an endometrial biopsy for purposes of diagnosing a luteal phase defect. Adequate progesterone production can be very easily diagnosed with a simple blood test. Even if there may be some rare individuals whose endometrium does not mature properly even with normal progesterone levels, the treatment is the same as that for patients who have unexplained infertility (Chapter 12). Therefore, there is really no need to have a biopsy. Furthermore, if you do have a biopsy and some treatment is initiated to correct a problem, a repeat biopsy to evaluate the effectiveness of that treatment is needed. Don't do it! Rather than having multiple biopsies to establish the diagnosis of luteal phase defect, serum progesterone levels can be used.

Thin Endometrium

The endometrium is another tissue that grows in response to estrogen. If the effect of estrogen is blocked, the endometrium may not develop adequately. This can sometimes occur as a result of the use of clomiphene. Normal endometrium usually develops to a thickness, as measured by ultrasound, of around ten millimeters. If it develops to only seven millimeters or less, pregnancy is extremely rare. The tissue just hasn't developed enough to allow it to accept a pregnancy. Endometrial development should be assessed by ultrasound in women on clomiphene, particularly if higher doses are being used, and any time gonadotropins are used.

Integrins

Integrins are proteins that are very "sticky." They play a role in the adhesion of one cell to the next and are important in the implantation process. Although a defect in their production appears to be a rare phenomenon, it apparently can occur. Assays for integrins may soon be available. This test does require an endometrial biopsy, and in couples with difficult unexplained infertility, this may be worthwhile.

CHAPTER ELEVEN
THE FEMALE AND OVULATION

In order to truly understand alterations and abnormalities of ovulation and the menstrual cycle, an understanding of the events that result in normal cyclic function is important. Following are several definitions, each of which will be discussed in more detail later in this chapter:

Day 1: the first day of *normal* flow of the menstrual period. In an *idealized* twenty-eight-day menstrual cycle, ovulation occurs on day fourteen.

    Follicular phase: the phase of the menstrual cycle beginning on day one and continuing until the time of ovulation.

    Proliferative phase: describes the development of the lining of the uterus. It occurs during, and is synchronous with, the follicular phase.

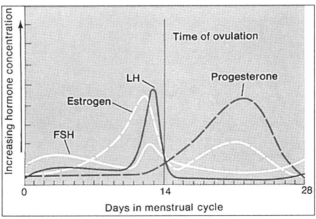

Reprinted with permission of The McGraw-Hill Companies from
Essentials of Human Anatomy & Physiology, 5E(1995), Hole J.

Luteal phase: the phase of the cycle beginning at the time of ovulation and continuing until the next menses begin.

Secretory phase: describes the changes that occur in the lining of the uterus after ovulation. It occurs during, and is synchronous with, the luteal phase.

Follicle: the fluid-filled sac that contains the developing egg and the cells surrounding that sac.

Estradiol: the primary estrogen produced by the developing follicle.

Corpus luteum: after release of the egg, the follicle becomes the corpus luteum and begins to produce progesterone.

Progesterone: the principal hormone produced by the corpus luteum.

OVERVIEW: FUNCTIONING OF THE OVARIES

At the time of puberty, the ovaries begin to function in a cyclic manner that results in menstrual cycles. This cyclic functioning of the ovaries results in the release of one egg per month, and the hormones associated with the development of that egg prime the rest of the reproductive system to allow, and then accept, a pregnancy should one occur. This cyclic functioning continues until menopause, at which time the development and release of eggs, and the production of the associated hormones, ceases.

The Ovarian Cycle: Follicular Phase

The ovarian cycle can be divided into two phases: the *follicular phase* and the *luteal phase*. It is during the follicular phase that the egg begins to develop and mature inside a fluid-filled sac within the ovary called the follicle. During its development, the follicle will increase in size from microscopic to two centimeters or more at the time of ovulation. Although only one egg is typically released each month, *many* eggs actually begin to develop. This development begins near the end of the previous menstrual cycle, even before the period has started. As these eggs continue to develop, fewer and fewer progress until only one remains. The remainder of the eggs that don't develop undergo a process known as *atresia* and are lost forever. The one egg that is destined to ovulate is usually "selected" as early as day five or six of the menstrual cycle. This follicle then continues to develop while the rest of the ones that had started to develop regress. The follicle in which this egg develops is primarily responsible for the production of estradiol, which is the principal hormone responsible for the development of the lining of the uterus, the changes in the cervical mucus, etc.

Egg and follicle development in the ovaries are under the control of a pituitary hormone known as FSH (follicle-stimulating hormone). Early in the follicular phase, FSH is produced by the pituitary in relatively large amounts, and this signals the eggs and their follicles to begin to develop. FSH continues to control the development of the egg(s) and follicle(s) throughout the follicular phase. When the one egg destined to ovulate has reached maturity and is ready to be ovulated, a second pituitary hormone known as LH (luteinizing hormone) triggers the release of the egg from the ovary. FSH primarily stimulates development and maturation of the follicles and eggs. LH primarily stimulates ovulation.

Luteal Phase

Once the egg has been released, the cells of the follicle that remain in the ovary quickly change and become known as the *corpus luteum*. The cells of the corpus luteum begin to produce significant amounts of progesterone in addition to estradiol. Progesterone induces the cells of the lining of the uterus to undergo the changes that will allow an embryo to implant and begin to grow. The life span of the corpus luteum is limited. Unless a pregnancy occurs and continues to stimulate it, the corpus luteum will produce progesterone for only twelve to fourteen days. As the corpus luteum begins to fail and progesterone production falls low enough, the cells of the lining of the uterus will begin to shed, a menstrual period begins, and the whole process starts over.

Of course, not all menstrual cycles are exactly twenty-eight days long. Cycles from twenty-six to thirty days or even longer may be normal. Normal ovulation occurs fourteen days before the onset of the next menstrual period. Therefore, in a thirty-two-day cycle, ovulation probably occurs on or about day eighteen. If a woman has regular menstrual cycles, she is in all probability ovulating. As we will see later, there are, however, instances in which bleeding can occur in the absence of ovulation, but this bleeding is typically very irregular and often abnormal in amount or duration.

OVARIAN RESERVES

A woman is born with all the eggs she will ever have—no new eggs are ever produced. With each menstrual cycle, some of these eggs are used up. There are always fewer and fewer eggs left in the ovary for each subsequent cycle. Furthermore, the healthiest and most responsive eggs are probably the first ones to be ovulated. In other words, when a woman is twenty, the eggs being released at that time are very fertile. By the time she reaches forty, the eggs remaining have been through as many as 350 cycles without ovulating—they just aren't as responsive to the stimulation from the pituitary hormones and have less fertility potential. With aging, the functioning of the ovaries declines and the capacity of the remaining eggs to establish a normal pregnancy decreases. Almost all of the decrease in female fertility with aging is due to this fact. This is known as *ovarian reserves.* How many functional eggs remain, and determination of ovarian reserves, is often important, particularly in older individuals.

Getting some idea of the extent of an individual's ovarian reserves can be a very important step in providing a couple with some idea about their chances for successful conception, especially before initiating expensive and time-consuming treatments. Both a day-three FSH level and a clomiphene citrate challenge test (see below) give us this information. After age thirty, and certainly after age thirty-five, these tests should be considered to be sure the ovaries are capable of producing adequate eggs, both in quantity and quality, before initiating some of the more expensive treatment alternatives.

PERSONAL STRATEGIES TO STRENGTHEN OVARIAN FUNCTION

There are a couple of things every woman can do to help ensure that her ovaries work to their maximal potential. First of all, *don't smoke.* There is excellent evidence that cigarette smoking not only makes it harder to get pregnant, but it also has a very deleterious effect on ovarian reserves. Women who smoke typically have far fewer functional eggs remaining in their ovaries than does someone their age who does not smoke. Secondly, watch your caffeine intake! Consuming more than the equivalent of a couple of cups of coffee per day has a negative effect on your chances of conceiving. Finally, if you are even considering getting pregnant, it is a good idea to take a prenatal or multivitamin. While this may not affect your chances of conceiving, it does help to decrease your risk of birth defects such as neural tube defects.

If you exercise on a regular basis, should you continue to do so if you are trying to get pregnant? For most individuals, the answer is "yes." Unless a woman exercises to an excessive level, there is no adverse effect of this activity. Women who train for and run marathons, or other elite types of athletes, may indeed experience changes in their menstrual cycles that make successful conception very difficult. If, however, you exercise three or four times a week just to stay in shape, continue to do so. It won't hurt your chances of getting pregnant and can be an excellent way to help you deal with the stress that the difficulty of getting pregnant may pose.

It is important to maintain your body weight in a normal range. Women who are too thin have a much higher incidence of ovulation problems. These can range from luteal phase defects to total absence of ovulation. By the same token, being excessively overweight can significantly interfere with normal egg production and ovulation.

Finally, maintain a positive attitude. There is no question this can be very difficult after dealing with all the frustration associated with trying to conceive. But you still need to try to do so. Remember, the treatment of impaired fertility is more successful than ever before, and the vast majority of couples can and will be successful in their pursuit. A positive attitude helps! There is good evidence that women who learn self-relaxation techniques or positive imaging techniques do better, and have higher success rates, than women who do not.

EVALUATION OF OVARIAN FUNCTION

Basal Body Temperatures (BBTs)

Recording basal body temperatures (BBTs) is often the first step in evaluating menstrual cycles. The detailed mechanics of proper BBT recording were discussed in Chapter 5. It involves taking your temperature every morning upon first awakening and before getting out of bed with a specially devised, very sensitive thermometer. Normal temperature charts are biphasic, with the temperature going up after ovulation as a result of progesterone. The BBT chart provides information about the length of the cycles, the regularity of the cycles, the timing of ovulation in those cycles and the length of the luteal phase. BBTs can also be very helpful in determining the adequacy of the timing of intercourse. Don't record temperature charts for more than a few months; if there is information to be gained from them, it will be apparent within that time. And don't try to interpret them yourself, particularly day to day. Either one of these things, let alone both, can make you crazy.

Progesterone Levels

Not all ovulations are the same. One woman may have twenty-eight-day cycles with ovulation on day fourteen and excellent progesterone production in the luteal phase, while another may have twenty-eight-day cycles with ovulation on day nineteen and very poor progesterone production. In other words, *having regular menstrual cycles means one is ovulating, but it doesn't necessarily mean she is ovulating well.* Temperature charts will provide some information about the adequacy of ovulation. Another more direct way to assess this is to measure progesterone levels in the blood in the middle of the luteal phase. Often a single, properly timed progesterone level will tell the physician a great deal about the adequacy of the cycle. A series of two or three progesterone levels obtained in the luteal phase is a very good way to assess the adequacy of the luteal phase.

Endometrial Biopsy

Another means by which the adequacy of a cycle may be assessed is by performing an endometrial biopsy in which a small piece of the lining of the uterus is removed from the uterus and examined microscopically. Endometrial biopsies are performed to diagnose a "luteal phase defect," a problem in which the cells of the lining of the uterus (the endometrium) do not properly undergo the series of changes that allow implantation to occur. This will be discussed further under luteal phase defect below, but for now suffice it to say that endometrial biopsies probably aren't necessary, since a serum progesterone will provide much the same information.

Pelvic Ultrasounds

Pelvic ultrasounds can be used to evaluate the development of the follicle (since it is fluid filled, it is easily seen on ultrasound). Ultrasounds are often used when any type of ovulation induction medication is taken, but may even be of some value in untreated cycles. Development of the follicle, the thickness of the endometrium and collapse of the follicle suggesting egg release can all be seen.

Measuring a Day-Three FSH

Measuring a day-three FSH and estradiol, and/or performing a clomiphene citrate challenge test provides information about a woman's ovarian reserves. As the number of eggs in the ovaries decreases, FSH levels rise as the pituitary attempts to further stimulate the ovaries in order to maintain regular ovulation and cycles. The FSH level on day three is very reflective of ovarian reserves—the fewer the number of eggs remaining in the ovaries, the higher the FSH level will be. Levels vary depending on the laboratory, but in general a day-three FSH level over fifteen, and certainly over twenty, suggests a very poor chance of conception.

Clomiphene Citrate Challenge Test

The clomiphene citrate challenge test involves checking FSH and estradiol levels on day three of the cycle, administering 100 milligrams of clomiphene citrate on days five through nine, and checking the FSH and progesterone levels on day ten. This test provides information that is even more reflective and reliable than the day-three FSH alone.

Prolactin

Prolactin is a pituitary hormone that functions primarily to stimulate breast milk production. However, even minor elevations of prolactin can alter the functioning of the ovary and result in abnormal cycles. Any woman with cycles that are anything but perfect should have a prolactin level checked.

TSH Levels

TSH (thyroid-stimulating hormone) is the hormone produced by the pituitary that controls the functioning of the thyroid gland. Alterations in thyroid function can have profound effects on ovarian function. Measuring TSH levels will detect an abnormality of thyroid function. Any woman with cycles that are anything but perfect should have a TSH level checked. Unless the TSH level is abnormal, there is no need to check any other thyroid test, as a sensitive TSH assay will reflect both hyper- and hypo-thyroid conditions.

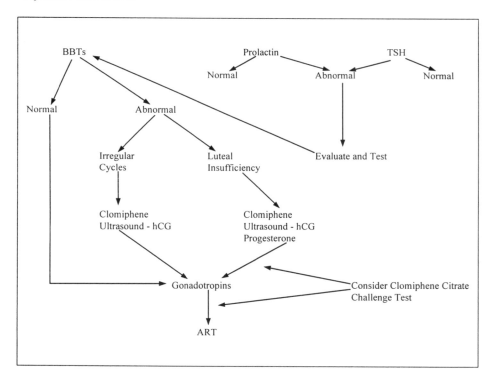

Treating Ovulation Disorders

Clomiphene Citrate

Clomiphene citrate (Clomid, Serophene) is the most commonly used medication for women with impaired fertility. Clomiphene is relatively inexpensive and is taken orally. Clomiphene "fools" the pituitary into thinking that the ovaries are not producing any estradiol by blocking the effect of estradiol on the pituitary. In other words, although there may still be plenty of estradiol around, the pituitary does not think so because it can't "see" it. The pituitary responds to this "apparently low estradiol level" by increasing the production of FSH, which in turn increases the stimulation to the ovary. In response to higher levels of FSH, the ovary becomes more likely to produce a mature egg.

Clomiphene is most useful in women with irregular, or even absent, ovulation. Clomiphene is typically given for five days beginning on either day four or day five of the cycle. The lowest dose of clomiphene is fifty milligrams, or one tablet. This should almost always be the starting dose. The response to clomiphene can be monitored with any combination of the tests mentioned above, including temperature charts, ultrasounds and progesterone levels. At the lower doses (fifty or 100 milligrams per day), simple recording of a BBT and a progesterone level in the mid-luteal phase are probably adequate. At higher doses (some physicians will use doses up to 250 milligrams), ultrasounds should be performed and hCG (see below) given if the follicle(s) has reached mature size. hCG functions as a signal to the follicle, just as LH does, that it is time to release the egg, or ovulate.

Side Effects of Clomiphene

Clomiphene is associated with a fair number of side effects. A small percentage of women will experience mild headaches, bloating, hot flashes or visual symptoms (you should notify your physician if you experience visual effects). A rather large percentage of couples report that the use of clomiphene results in some emotional instability. If you are taking clomiphene and find that your emotions are a little hard to control, especially in the second half of the cycle, blame it on the clomiphene.

There are no known risks to the fetus or adverse effects on the infant should conception occur. Ovarian cysts may occur in some individuals on clomiphene, but if no additional clomiphene is given, the cysts will almost always resolve on their own. For this reason a pelvic exam or an ultrasound should be performed between cycles of clomiphene to be sure the ovaries have returned to normal before more clomiphene is taken. There is some increase in the risk of multiple pregnancies with clomiphene. Women who conceive have about a seven percent chance of twins. The risk of triplets, quadruplets, etc. is not really increased.

Other Considerations Concerning Clomiphene

Either a dose works, or it doesn't. If taking fifty milligrams a day does not result in normalization of ovulation (and therefore your cycle) one month, there is no point in trying that dose again. The dose needs to be increased the next month.

More is worse, not better. Once the dose that normalizes the cycle and results in good ovulation and progesterone production is determined, there is no point in increasing the dose further. In fact, increasing the dose further may actually make it harder or even impossible to get pregnant. Remember: Clomiphene functions by preventing the pituitary from "seeing" the estradiol that is present. It does the same thing to the cells that produce the cervical mucus and to the cells that line the uterus—if they don't "see" the estradiol, the cells of the cervix won't produce the mucus, or the cells lining the uterus won't develop to an extent adequate to allow implantation. Everyone has a threshold dose of clomiphene (the dose that normalizes ovulation). Going beyond that dose does more harm than good.

Clomiphene is an antiestrogen. This means that it does indeed prevent some cells from "seeing" the estradiol and because of this blocks the action of estradiol on those cells. The possibility of this type of effect needs to be checked once the threshold dose is achieved. This should include a post-coital test to be sure that there is adequate cervical mucus production, and a measurement of the thickness of the endometrium by ultrasound to be sure that it is developing to an adequate thickness. Normal endometrium develops to about ten millimeters in thickness; an endometrial thickness of seven millimeters or less is associated with very poor pregnancy rates. This is often a problem at some of the higher doses of clomiphene— although it results in ovulation, there is enough of an antiestrogen effect on the cervical mucus or endometrium to prevent pregnancy from occurring even though ovulation is normalized.

The vast majority of the pregnancies that occur as the result of the use of clomiphene occur within the first four ovulatory cycles. Once the threshold dose is achieved, there is really little point in pursuing the use of clomiphene beyond four, or certainly six, cycles at most. (The chances of conceiving in a cycle of clomiphene beyond the fourth may be as low as three to four percent, and decrease even further soon thereafter.) There is another reason for limiting the number of cycles of clomiphene. There is at least one study suggesting that the use of clomiphene for more than a year is associated with an increase in the risk of ovarian cancer.

Finally, and perhaps most importantly, there is no role for clomiphene in a woman with regular ovulatory cycles. There is absolutely no good evidence that clomiphene improves pregnancy rates in women with normal cycles. It is not a "fertility enhancer" and, in fact, because of its anti-estrogen properties, it can actually make it harder to get pregnant rather than easier.

Progesterone

Progesterone is often used by itself or in conjunction with other ovulation-induction medications. Administering progesterone during the luteal phase directly increases the progesterone level. It is often used when there is concern about a possible abnormal luteal phase or luteal phase defect. Only progesterone, the same hormone produced by the body, should be used. The use of natural progesterone has not been associated with any risk of abnormality of the child. There are many progestins, or progesterone-like medications available, but many of these have been associated with birth defects. As far as anyone knows, pure progesterone is perfectly safe to use.

hCG

In "nature's way," the pituitary produces large amounts of LH when the follicle is mature and the egg is ready to be released. This LH "surge" induces the final changes that result in egg release. hCG is a hormone produced by the placenta during pregnancy. Its structure is remarkably similar to LH, and the ovary really can't tell the difference between the two hormones. We can, therefore, use hCG to mimic the actions of LH. (Preparations of pure LH are not yet available.) When other ovulation medications are used, such as higher doses of clomiphene or the gonadotropins, the pituitary is no longer capable of adequately signaling the ovary with an LH "surge." This signal must therefore be provided, and we do so by administering hCG. In most cases, ovulation will occur thirty-six to forty hours after the administration of hCG.

Smaller doses of hCG are often given during the luteal phase. These smaller doses of hCG provide stimulation to the corpus luteum to make progesterone. If luteal phase hCG is being used, one must be somewhat careful about the timing of a pregnancy test—pregnancy tests detect the presence of hCG, and doing the test too early will simply detect the hCG that was administered.

THE GONADOTROPINS: PERGONAL, METRODIN, HUMEGON, FERTINEX, FOLLISTIM AND GONAL-F

Pergonal, Metrodin, Humegon, Fertinex, Follistim and Gonal-F are collectively known as gonadotropins. Pergonal and Humegon are formulations of LH and FSH, while Metrodin, Fertinex, Follistim and Gonal-F are FSH alone. For purposes of discussion, these hormonal preparations can be grouped together as the "gonadotropins." There is very little difference in their action, and they can essentially be used interchangeably.

The gonadotropins function by directly stimulating the ovaries. The pituitary normally produces FSH and LH to stimulate the ovaries; by using the gonadotropins, this level of stimulation is directly increased.

Gonadotropins can be used alone or in combination with a GnRH agonist (see below). Administration is begun between day three and five of the cycle and usually continued for a total of five to nine days depending upon the response. One of the primary goals of gonadotropin therapy is to induce multiple-egg development. The ovulation of multiple eggs and the resulting production of higher hormone levels explain the conception rates associated with the use of gonadotropins. Whereas the use of clomiphene typically results in the production of only one or two eggs, gonadotropins can induce any number of eggs to develop, from a couple all the way to thirty or more. Their use must, therefore, be carefully monitored and supervised by a physician familiar and comfortable with their use.

Monitoring Gonadotropins

The response to the gonadotropins is usually monitored with a combination of estradiol levels and pelvic ultrasounds. The ultrasounds allow the physician to see the number of follicles and eggs that are developing. When a follicle reaches a certain size, around eighteen millimeters in diameter, the likelihood is greatest that the egg contained therein is mature. Thus, we can get not only a good indication as to the maturity of the follicles and eggs, but ultrasounds also provide a very clear picture of how many are mature and capable of ovulation. The estradiol levels also give some indication as to the health and well-being of the developing follicles. When the follicles are mature size, hCG is given and ovulation will occur thirty-six to forty hours later.

In contradistinction to clomiphene which works by "tricking" the pituitary to increase its stimulation of the ovaries, the gonadotropins act *directly* on the ovaries. Rather than any type of antiestrogen effect, therefore, estradiol levels and the effects of estradiol are actually dramatically increased with the gonadotropins. For example, the gonadotropins enhance rather than impair cervical mucus production.

Risk Factors of Gonadotropins

There are relatively few side effects associated with the gonadotropins. Aside from the emotional roller coaster that all couples experience while attempting to conceive, there are no significant emotional side effects associated with the menotropins. The two most frequent problems are enlarged ovaries and multiple births. It is normal for the ovaries to be enlarged after the use of the gonadotropins; we have, after all induced three or four (and sometimes more) eggs to develop and ovulate. Most of the symptoms associated with this enlargement occur after ovulation, during the luteal phase when three or four corpora lutea (plural of corpus luteum) are actively producing progesterone. Simply decreasing one's activity level is all that is usually necessary. In more severe cases, hyperstimulation may occur.

Multiple Pregnancies. Anyone initiating treatment with the gonadotropins must realize that multiple pregnancy is a possibility. Twin pregnancies occur as frequently as twenty percent of the time in women who conceive on gonadotropins. And everyone has heard the stories of women who have conceived far more than twins. However, higher order multiple pregnancies (triplets or more) don't have to be a significant risk to women on gonadotropins. Remember, the response to the gonadotropins is monitored with ultrasound. The number of follicles and eggs that are developing can be seen prior to giving hCG to trigger ovulation. If an unacceptable number of follicles develops, we simply don't give the hCG; ovulation doesn't occur and the cycle is wasted, but a canceled cycle is better than a litter! There is no hard and fast number that constitutes an acceptable number of follicles. That depends on many factors including the number of previous attempts, age and other factors involved. This is why one should have an expert monitoring their cycle, so these types of information can be considered and carefully thought out decisions made.

Ovarian Cancer. There has been some concern raised that the use of the gonadotropins is associated with an increased risk of developing ovarian cancer. This issue has been very carefully evaluated, and the data does not support such an association. It does seem that there may be a group of women with ovulatory dysfunction who are at increased risk of developing ovarian cancer with or without treatment. However, for the average women using gonadotropins, there is no evidence that this use is associated with an increased risk of ovarian cancer.

Other Considerations

The two major drawbacks to the gonadotropins are expense and the fact that they must be administered by injection. These hormones are very expensive, and one cycle can cost as much as $1,000 or more. Pergonal, Humegon, and Metrodin are given intramuscularly in the hip. We usually teach the husband to administer these shots. Fertinex, Follistim, and Gonal-F are given subcutaneously and can most often be self-administered.

Follistim and Gonal-F are the most recently approved gonadotropins. These two hormone preparations are produced by recombinant DNA technology, meaning that they are produced in the laboratory rather than isolated from human urine. They are purer preparations of FSH.

There is little if any reason to record a BBT chart while on the gonadotropins. All of the other monitoring provides more than enough information about the cycle. Progesterone levels are also checked during the luteal phase, and the length of the luteal phase is easily determined since the time of ovulation is known. All of this data provides more than enough information about the adequacy of the cycle.

The gonadotropins should only be used every other month at most. It is simply too much for the ovaries to use them every month; the ovaries need at least a month in between to recover. There is a lot of debate as to what is the maximal number of cycles one should attempt with the menotropins. Much of this will depend on a number of considerations that were discussed in Chapter 6, but suffice it to say that the chances of successful conception make it hard to justify more than three attempts in most situations. If conception has not occurred within three attempts, an ART procedure should be considered.

GnRH Agonists

GnRH is a hormone produced by the hypothalamus. The hypothalamus is "control central." It controls many of the basal functions of the body, including reproduction. It controls reproduction by controlling the production and release of LH and FSH from the pituitary. GnRH agonists, such as leuprolide acetate (Lupron) and nafarelin acetate (Synarel), very selectively inhibit the ability of the pituitary to produce and release LH and FSH. If LH and FSH aren't produced, the ovaries are not stimulated. In other words, by using Lupron we can temporarily "turn off" the ovaries.

There is a good rationale for doing this, for "turning off" the ovaries before we begin to stimulate them with the gonadotropins. Remember that egg development for the upcoming cycle actually begins late in the previous cycle. The timing of the beginning of this development varies, but progesterone usually suppresses this development until late in the luteal phase. In some women, particularly those who produce relatively low levels of progesterone, the development of the eggs for the next cycle may begin too early. If the gonadotropins are begun on day five, the development may have already progressed far enough that the goal of gonadotropin therapy, i.e., improved quantity and quality of follicles, is unattainable. When the GnRh agonists are used, complete suppression is achieved. Thus, when the gonadotropins are begun, we are starting with a "clean slate." No follicle and egg development has occurred, and stimulating and controlling their development from the very beginning is possible.

The ovaries are most easily suppressed by beginning the GnRH agonist in the luteal phase, usually about day twenty-one. This does imply, silly as it may sound, that you should not attempt pregnancy in a month in which you anticipate starting a GnRH agonist on day twenty-one. There are a fairly large number of cases in which an agonist has been started and a pregnancy has occurred, and there do not appear to be any adverse effects. However, why chance it? After starting the agonist on day twenty-one, the next period will probably be relatively normal and will probably occur on time. An ultrasound is performed soon thereafter, and if the ovaries have been suppressed, the gonadotropins are begun. Using a GnRH agonist in conjunction with the gonadotropins has several advantages:

- Premature ovulation will not occur. Ovulation will occur about forty hours after the administration of hCG.
- The follicles and eggs that do develop in response to the gonado-tropins are more synchronous in their development. Their maturity levels are about the same.
- It may be far easier to get more than one follicle to develop by adding a GnRH agonist than it is with the gonadotropins alone.
- Luteal phase progesterone, both in terms of levels and duration of production, is improved.

There are several indications for adding a GnRH agonist to the gonadotropins. A history of premature ovulation, difficulty getting more than one follicle to develop, and poor progesterone levels or short luteal phases while on the gonadotropins alone suggest that a GnRH agonist would be worthwhile. The combination of a GnRH agonist and gonadotropins is often more effective in correcting a significant luteal phase insufficiency than are gonadotropins alone.

The GnRH agonists are administered either by subcutaneous injection (Lupron) or by nasal spray (Synarel). When used for this purpose, they have few if any side effects. Addition of a GnRH agonist does usually result in the need for additional gonadotropins to achieve adequate ovarian stimulation.

PARLODEL AND DOSTINEX

Parlodel and Dostinex are medications that specifically and effectively decrease the production of prolactin from the pituitary. As noted above, prolactin levels should be checked in anyone with cycles that are anything but perfectly normal. If the prolactin level is above fifty, some radiological evaluation should be performed prior to initiating treatment to see if a pituitary microadenoma is present (these are benign tumors in the pituitary that produce prolactin). Treatment with Parlodel and Dostinex should be initiated and adjusted until the prolactin level is back in the normal range. Nausea, which is one of the more common side effects of Parlodel, can be avoided by simply placing the tablet in the vagina rather than swallowing it.

LUTEAL PHASE INSUFFICIENCY

There are some women who, although they may ovulate regularly, do not produce adequate progesterone or who produce progesterone for a shorter period of time than they should. This results in the lining of the uterus receiving inadequate stimulation or support to undergo the series of changes necessary to allow implantation to occur. Thus, although conception may occur, pregnancy does not because of failure to implant.

There are several factors associated with luteal phase insufficiency, including a low percent body fat, elevated prolactin levels and even stress. Luteal phase insufficiency can be diagnosed by checking progesterone levels in the mid-luteal phase, by careful evaluation of BBTs and bleeding patterns or by endometrial biopsies. I do not believe in endometrial biopsies for this purpose. They are invasive, potentially painful, costly and unnecessary. Progesterone levels and BBTs will provide adequate information about the luteal phase in most women. If these are adequate, there are very few women indeed for whom an endometrial biopsy will reveal a problem.

This approach of not doing endometrial biopsies may miss a small percentage of women in whom only the endometrial biopsy would reveal an abnormality. However, the approach to treatment for these women will be the same if we do a biopsy and reveal an abnormality as it would be for women with unexplained infertility. We would initiate the same treatment whether or not we have the results of an endometrial biopsy. So why do it? This group of women with possible luteal phase insufficiency should just be treated like women with unexplained infertility. In other words, if the treatment is going to be the same anyhow, why not just proceed with that treatment rather than performing a lot of testing that is not going to change the treatment.

Luteal phase insufficiency can be treated with progesterone suppositories, low-dose clomiphene given on days three through seven, hCG at the time of follicular maturity or a combination of any or all of these. If this is unsuccessful, combined GnRH agonist and gonadotropin therapy seems to be far more effective in correcting luteal phase insufficiency than are gonadotropins alone.

HYPERSTIMULATION

Ovarian hyperstimulation syndrome (OHSS) is a syndrome that can occur in the luteal phase following the use of gonadotropins (and rarely after clomiphene). Following the development of multiple follicles, multiple corpora lutea develop. As a result of this, the ovaries enlarge, usually to an insignificant level but sometimes to as much as eight or ten centimeters or more. The extent of enlargement is proportional to the number of corpora lutea present and can be somewhat predicted by the level of estradiol prior to hCG administration at the time of ovulation. Most women on gonado-tropins will experience some symptoms of hyperstimulation with bloating and some ovarian tenderness being common. These symptoms are usually mild—you may want to wear baggy sweat pants rather tight jeans and may not feel like going to aerobics class. But usually normal activity can be pursued. More severe hyperstimulation is uncommon and is more likely to occur when these medications are intentionally used to achieve the development of more than just a few follicles (such as in an ART procedure). In severe hyperstimulation, the ovaries are very enlarged, and fluid may accumulate in the abdominal cavity. Women may experience bloating, difficulty breathing, weight gain and decreased urine output. Although unusual, this can require hospitalization for management until the ovaries begin to return to normal size. If a woman does not conceive in a cycle using gonadotropins, the ovaries will return to normal quickly after the period begins. If pregnancy does occur, it may take several weeks for the ovaries to return to their normal size.

POLYCYSTIC OVARIES

A special subset of ovulatory abnormalities is known as polycystic ovary syndrome, or PCOS. There are many variants of PCOS, and the process can be mild to very severe, but virtually all women with PCOS have a history of irregular menstrual periods, usually since the time of puberty. The menstrual cycles are irregular because women with this process ovulate very irregularly, and in some cases not at all. Other symptoms or signs that may be associated with this process include infertility, excessive hair growth and obesity.

It is not known what causes some women to develop PCOS. There is evidence that some individuals may inherit the process from their mothers, but for most individuals the events that result in the development of this process are unknown. We do know, however, that virtually every woman with PCOS has elevated insulin levels in her blood, and it is felt that these insulin levels may be directly responsible for the abnormalities seen in PCOS. In fact, there is some evidence that exposure to high insulin levels at the time of puberty may result in the development of PCOS.

Once this process gets initiated, the regular cyclic events that result in normal menstrual cycles do not occur. Rather, PCOS is characterized by a very constant hormone picture day after day. The pituitary produces higher levels of LH than are found in normally cycling women. The ovary responds to this higher-than-normal level of LH by producing higher-than-normal levels of male hormones, specifically testosterone. (This is exactly what the ovaries are supposed to do in response to high levels of LH. The higher-than-normal levels of testosterone are responsible for the increased hair growth which is often noted.) The testosterone is then converted by other tissues, specifically the fat cells, into estrogen. The hypothalamus then "sees" the high levels of estrogen and responds perfectly normally by telling the pituitary to produce more LH and less FSH. The pituitary produces more LH, and the whole thing becomes a vicious cycle. In addition, the lower-than-normal levels of FSH decrease the stimulation to the ovary that is needed in order for an egg to mature to the point where it can be ovulated. In other words, every part of the system is responding appropriately to the signals it is receiving; it's just that somewhere along the line something got mixed up. A vicious cycle is established and will continue until something happens to break the cycle.

Diagnosing PCOS is pretty straightforward. If a woman has a life-long history of irregular periods, she probably has PCOS. It is not necessary to have blood drawn for LH and FSH levels to diagnose this process; the history is good enough. If excess hair growth is present, the physician may want to check a testosterone and DHEA-S level just to be sure there is no tumor producing those hormones. If a pelvic ultrasound is performed, it will reveal many small (rarely more than a few millimeters in diameter) cysts in the ovaries. These are small follicular cysts that have begun development but have not progressed beyond this size because of the relative lack of FSH.

For women who do not want to be pregnant, birth control pills are an excellent means of managing PCOS. The birth control pills suppress LH, thereby suppressing the ovaries and decreasing their production of hormones, including testosterone. Birth control pills also result in normalization of the periods.

Clomiphene was designed for use in women with PCOS. Clomiphene prevents the pituitary from "seeing" the amount of estrogen that is present. If the pituitary doesn't "see" any estrogen, it responds by decreasing the production of LH and increasing the production of FSH. This is exactly what is needed—this is one way to break the cycle. If the FSH levels are increased enough, the ovary will respond by maturing one or more eggs and ovulation will occur. As many as ninety percent of women with PCOS will ovulate in response to clomiphene, with about half that many becoming successfully pregnant.

There are, however, certainly individuals with PCOS in whom clomiphene is unsuccessful; in spite of maximal doses of clomiphene, ovulation does not occur. These individuals are then candidates for ovulation induction using gonadotropins, either alone or in combination with a GnRH agonist. This can be somewhat tricky. Remember, there are lots of little follicles sitting in the ovaries just waiting for some FSH to come along. Women with PCOS are at increased risk for producing large numbers of eggs in response to the gonadotropins, and consequently their risk for ovarian hyperstimulation is also increased. This excessive ovarian response can be managed by performing an ART procedure, which gives the physician the opportunity to remove all of the eggs, and return only the number appropriate for an individual of that age. Thus the risk of multiple pregnancies can be safely controlled.

There are also surgical approaches for dealing with PCOS. The earliest treatment of PCOS was, in fact, a surgical procedure known as a *wedge resection,* in which a significant part of the ovary was removed. This procedure worked because it broke the cycle by decreasing the amount of testosterone produced from the ovaries. It is, however, rarely performed anymore because of the need for major surgery, the risk of formation of scar tissue after this procedure, and the availability of medical therapies. There are, however, laparoscopic procedures in which much the same thing is accomplished—part of the ovary is destroyed. The risk of forming scar tissue after a laparoscopic procedure for PCOS is significant. Furthermore, any type of procedure in which part of the ovary is destroyed results in temporary improvement only. Eventually the PCOS pattern will return. Surgical therapy is, therefore, usually reserved for individuals whose PCOS cannot be managed with the medical therapies listed above.

One of the most exciting developments in the area of PCOS is an increased awareness of the role of elevated insulin levels in this process. There are medications available (e.g., Rezulin, Glucophage) for the treatment of adult-onset diabetes mellitus that specifically reduce insulin levels in the blood. Preliminary studies have demonstrated that insulin levels in individuals with PCOS can also be reduced by using these medications. These studies have also demonstrated that, by reducing insulin levels, many of the abnormalities of PCOS can be reversed and in many cases the ovaries will begin to function normally. In virtually all women with PCOS treated with insulin-lowering agents, ovarian function is improved. Although further study and evaluation of these agents is needed (and these studies are currently underway in our center as well as others), they hold *great* promise, and they may well be the way PCOS is managed and treated in the near future.

CHAPTER TWELVE
UNEXPLAINED INFERTILITY

OVERVIEW

Testing and evaluation will demonstrate one or more causes of decreased fertility in the vast majority of couples. There are, however, still a significant number of couples in whom no demonstrable problems exist. This percentage will vary depending on the approach used, but is usually somewhere around fifteen percent. Some of the more recent advances, including sperm function testing, will undoubtedly decrease this number even further. But there will always be many couples in whom the problem remains unidentified. There is, for example, no test to evaluate whether or not the fallopian tubes function appropriately in terms of egg pickup. The tubes can certainly be assessed visually by hysterosalpingogram, by laparoscopy, and even by salpingoscopy, but none of these tests tell us whether or not the tubes will seek out, pick up and transport an egg when the ovary releases it.

DIAGNOSIS

The diagnosis of unexplained infertility can be a difficult one for a couple to reconcile. It is very frustrating to go through months or even years of extensive testing and treatment and still not know what the problem is. It is much easier to hear "this is what the problem is, and this is what we can do to fix it," than it is to hear "we don't know what is wrong." However, while it can be psychologically very difficult not to know the answer, from a medical and treatment standpoint, it is not bad at all. The treatment of couples with unexplained infertility is pretty straightforward, and the success rates are very high.

As mentioned above, the percentage of couples who have unexplained infertility depends on the approach used to evaluate their potential problems. If, for example, a physician does a laparoscopy on every woman, the percentage of couples with unexplained infertility may be relatively low since the physician may diagnose mild endometriosis in a significant number of these women. By the same token, if a physician does endometrial biopsies on every woman, the percentage of couples with unexplained infertility may be lower because a certain number will be diagnosed as having a luteal phase defect.

However, diagnosing and treating mild endometriosis does not improve conception rates (Chapter 9). And we have already discussed the fact that the treatment for a luteal phase defect is the same as it is for a couple with unexplained infertility. So why not do this: Avoid the laparoscopy and the endometrial biopsy, and proceed with treatment just as we would for any couple with otherwise unexplained infertility. Admittedly, there will be couples in this group with mild endometriosis or luteal phase defects, but it doesn't matter! *The treatment of these couples will be the same whether we make those diagnoses or not.* And we have avoided costly, invasive and painful procedures.

TREATMENT

There are certainly some tests that need to be done before assigning a couple to this category. We do need to be sure that the semen analysis, post-coital test and sperm function tests are normal. We need to know that there is no evidence of prior infection or surgery and that the uterus and fallopian tubes are normal. We need to know the ovaries appear normal by ultrasound and that the pelvic exam is okay. And we need to know that ovulation occurs with adequate progesterone production and adequate luteal phase length by BBTs. We don't need to know anything else.

The algorithm for unexplained infertility is presented below. As discussed in Chapter 6, exactly how this algorithm is followed depends on a lot of considerations that individualize this approach for each couple and their particular circumstances.

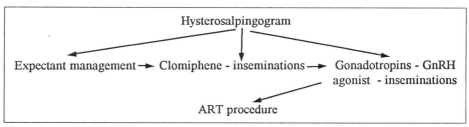

**Unexplained Infertility/Endometriosis Without Anatomic Distortion
Luteal Phase Insufficiency**

Hysterosalpingogram

By the time the hysterosalpingogram is performed, all of the evaluation mentioned above, with the exception of the sperm function testing, should be complete. The appropriate timing for the performance of sperm function testing remains to be determined as it is such a relatively new test, but it should certainly be considered before proceeding to an ART procedure, if not earlier. A hysterosalpingogram performed with oil-soluble contrast material improves conception rates for the next several months after it is done. Taking into account all other considerations, it may be very reasonable to simply attempt conception without intervention for a while (known as *expectant management*) after undergoing an HSG. If this doesn't work within four to six months at most, it is time to move on and consider more aggressive treatment.

Clomiphene

The role of clomiphene in the treatment of unexplained infertility is very controversial. The use of clomiphene, particularly for the treatment of a suspected luteal phase defect, is worthwhile. Luteal phase defects can be very adequately treated with the use of clomiphene (started on day three of the cycle), hCG and progesterone suppositories. This is certainly a treatment alternative in which all considerations must be taken into account. As with any treatment alternative, the chances of success must be balanced against all other considerations. For a twenty-five-year-old couple with a year and a half of infertility, this step probably makes sense. For a couple who is forty with a year and half of infertility, it probably doesn't make sense. For this couple, the chances of success simply don't justify the amount of time that would be spent pursuing this alternative. A more aggressive alternative with a greater chance of success would be a better option. If clomiphene treatment is pursued, do so for four months at most. If it hasn't worked by then, it is time to try something else.

This is one group, particularly when the female is over age thirty and certainly when she is over age thirty-five, where determination of ovarian reserves is probably indicated. As discussed in detail in Chapter 11, as a woman ages, the quantity of eggs remaining in the ovaries declines. And as the quantity declines, so does the capacity of any of those remaining eggs to successfully establish a pregnancy. Doing a clomiphene citrate challenge test, to be certain that the ovaries are capable of functioning adequately, is a reasonable step. It is easy, inexpensive and noninvasive, and it can provide very valuable information before embarking on more expensive treatment options. As many as ten percent of women over age thirty-five may have compromised ovarian reserves, and that percentage increases even further as one gets older.

Gonadotropins

Superovulation with gonadotropins is a worthwhile step in this algorithm for the majority of couples. Whether or not inseminations are performed is also somewhat debatable, but the predominance of evidence suggests that pregnancy rates are slightly higher if inseminations are performed than if intercourse occurs. With all the injections, expense of the medications and the inconvenience of the monitoring, if there is even a suggestion that inseminations improve the chances of success, they would seem to be worthwhile. If this step is not successful within two or three attempts, consider moving on to one of the ART procedures.

The vast majority of couples with unexplained infertility will conceive. It is a hard diagnosis to deal with psychologically. There are diagnoses that are much harder to deal with medically.

Chapter Thirteen
The ART Procedures

ART stands for Assisted Reproductive Technology, and it is the group of procedures that falls under this heading that have revolutionized the entire approach to couples with impaired fertility. These procedures offer couples opportunities to conceive (where only a few years ago they may have had no chance whatsoever) with success rates that exceed any other procedure or technique available. In this chapter we will examine each and every one of these procedures in detail.

IVF stands for *in vitro fertilization*, commonly known as *test tube babies*. IVF is the grandfather of all of these procedures. Louise Brown, the first child conceived as a result of IVF, was born in 1981 as the result of years of research and effort by Drs. Steptoe and Edwards. The seventeen years since this initial success have witnessed a virtual explosion of information relating to, and understanding of, this procedure. There are now over two hundred IVF programs in this country alone, and tens of thousands of couples have conceived healthy children as a result of IVF procedures.

GIFT is the acronym for *gamete intrafallopian transfer*. GIFT was developed a few years after IVF and entails placing unfertilized eggs and sperm directly into the fallopian tubes.

ZIFT is the acronym for *zygote intrafallopian transfer*. ZIFT is sort of a hybrid of GIFT and IVF in that fertilization of the eggs occurs in the laboratory, but then the newly fertilized eggs, or zygotes, are placed back into the fallopian tubes rather than into the uterus as they would be in IVF.

ICSI is the acronym for *intracytoplasmic sperm injection*. ICSI is a micromanipulation technique whereby a single sperm is injected into an egg.

This technique may be used in conjunction with either IVF or ZIFT and offers fertility to men with extremely compromised sperm counts.

INDUCING OVULATION

It is important to remember that in "nature's way" only one egg reaches maturity and is released each cycle. Louise Brown was conceived this way, by using the one egg her mother naturally produced. But it quickly became apparent that if more than one egg could be produced, the chances of the procedure working were much better. Ovulation induction, or getting more than one healthy egg to be produced, is now an integral part of each and every one of the ART procedures. There are many techniques available to accomplish this, and in large part they are similar to the ones previously described (see Chapter 10). There is, however, one approach that has achieved overwhelming popularity and has demonstrated the greatest success—the combination of GnRH agonists and gonadotropins (Pergonal, Metrodin, Humegon, Fertinex, Gonal-F and Follistim). It is this approach that will be explained in detail, and it is the same regardless of which of the ART procedures is being anticipated.

The rationale behind the use of GnRH agonists in addition to gonadotropins is explained in detail in Chapter 11. In essence, this combination allows the physician to induce the ovaries to produce multiple oocytes of similar maturity with minimal if any risk of premature ovulation. This is far and away the most commonly used, and most successful, combination for ovulation induction in anticipation of an ART procedure.

The ovaries are most easily suppressed by beginning the GnRH agonist in the middle of the luteal phase, usually about day twenty-one. This does imply that, as silly as it may sound, you should not attempt pregnancy in a month in which you anticipate starting a GnRH agonist on day twenty-one. There are a fairly large number of cases in which an agonist has been started and a pregnancy has occurred, and there do not appear to be any adverse effects. However, why chance it? After starting the agonist on day twenty-one, the next period should begin on time. If it doesn't, contact your physician.

Once the period begins, an ultrasound is performed and an estradiol checked to ensure that ovarian suppression has been achieved. The gonadotropins, which must be given by injection, are then begun and continued for a total of eight to ten days. The dose of the gonadotropins is individualized, but the goal is the development of multiple follicles. When gonadotropins are used for ovulation induction and inseminations, the goal is the development of just a few follicles. When gonadotropins are used for an ART procedure, the goal is the development of multiple follicles. For purposes of discussion, let's say that we would like ten follicles to develop.

The response to the gonadotropins is monitored with a combination of ultrasounds and estradiol levels. While these certainly don't need to be performed every day, the monitoring must be frequent enough that the physician can determine when the follicles are mature. While the eggs themselves can't be seen by ultrasound, the follicles are easily visualized. When a follicle reaches a certain size, the likelihood of there being a mature and healthy egg within that follicle is maximal. Parameters vary somewhat among physicians, but a follicular diameter of eighteen millimeters is commonly used as suggesting maturity. When the follicles reach a mature size, hCG is given (hCG induces the final maturation and egg release). Approximately forty hours after hCG, ovulation will occur. With the use of a GnRH agonist in addition to the gonadotropins, premature ovulation, or ovulation significantly before forty hours after hCG, is very rare. Therefore, egg retrieval, the process of actually removing the eggs from the ovaries, is scheduled between thirty-four and thirty-six hours after hCG, thus ensuring that the eggs will be mature but will not yet have been released from the ovaries.

There is another means of inducing ovulation for ART procedures that has also been successful. This technique has been used for individuals who are defined as low responders—individuals whose ovaries do not respond to the standard ovulation induction technique with production of as many eggs as would have been expected. In this approach, a standard low-dose oral contraceptive (OCP) is begun with the menses the month before the anticipated cycle and taken for twenty-one days. Beginning on the third day after discontinuation of the OCPs, Lupron is administered in very small, microgram amounts (twenty to forty twice a day). Stimulation with gonadotropins is then begun on the third day of Lupron administration at a dosage of 225 units twice daily. Monitoring is then performed as with the standard protocol, and stimulation is continued until follicular maturity.

Retrieving the Eggs

There are two approaches used for egg retrieval: the vaginal approach using ultrasound guidance and the laparoscopic approach. The vaginal approach is used for IVF procedures and for the first part of the ZIFT procedure, while a GIFT procedure is done laparoscopically.

Egg retrieval by the vaginal approach is accomplished with the use of a vaginal ultrasound and a long needle that can be precisely guided into each follicle within the ovary. The ovaries typically sit right at the top of the vagina, and the needle is simply placed through the wall of the vagina and into the ovaries; it doesn't go through the uterus or through the fallopian tubes. Each individual follicle is visualized, and the needle inserted into the follicle. A small amount of suction is then applied to the needle, and the contents of each follicle aspirated into a test tube. The test tube is then transferred to the laboratory personnel who examine the contents of the tube microscopically, isolate any eggs contained therein, evaluate them and place them in an incubator.

General anesthesia for vaginal egg retrieval is not required. Vaginal egg retrieval can be performed under sedation in an operating room setting, or in an office-type setting with simple use of oral pain medications. The latter approach is becoming increasingly more common because of the cost savings associated with this approach. A typical retrieval takes no more than ten to fifteen minutes. Some women may experience mild cramping after a vaginal egg retrieval, but most resume normal activity the same day of the procedure. While there are risks to any type of operative procedure, the risks associated with vaginal egg retrieval, including bleeding, infection and damage to organs are absolutely minimal.

The whole goal of IVF is to achieve fertilization and early embryo development in the laboratory. Every step of this process must, therefore, mimic as closely as possible the environment that would normally exist in the fallopian tube. Embryo culturing (achieving the fertilization of eggs and early development of embryos) requires meticulous preparation of carefully designed media (the fluid in which the embryos will be maintained in the laboratory), the use of controlled environments within incubators and painstaking attention to detail.

ART PROCEDURES
IVF (In Vitro Fertilization)

Following retrieval, a sperm sample is obtained from the husband. After preparation of the sperm sample, a small quantity of sperm (50,000-100,000) is added to the dish containing each egg, and incubation continues. After fourteen to eighteen hours, the eggs are reevaluated because if fertilization has occurred, evidence of this will be present at this point. Eggs that have been fertilized but have not yet begun to divide are known as zygotes. The zygotes are returned to the incubators, and culture continues for an additional couple of days. During this period, cell division begins, and after a total of approximately seventy-two hours, the embryos typically have developed to about the eight- to ten-cell stage.

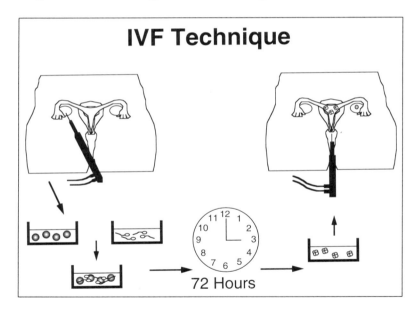

IVF Technique

72 Hours

We currently perform embryo transfers at approximately seventy-two hours after egg retrieval, but transfers can be performed anywhere from twenty-four to ninety-six hours or more after egg retrieval. An appropriate number of embryos are loaded into a small plastic catheter. This catheter is gently inserted through the cervix and into the uterine cavity where the embryos are deposited. This is a painless procedure that requires no anesthesia and takes just minutes, although it is often suggested that the patient remain lying down for a while after embryo transfer. Minimal activity the day of the transfer is suggested, but after that, normal activity may be resumed. Two weeks later, a pregnancy test can be performed.

IVF was initially developed as a means of bypassing the fallopian tubes; the events that normally occur in the fallopian tubes such as fertilization and early development occur instead in the laboratory, and the embryos are then placed directly into the uterus. The most obvious indication for IVF is damaged, absent or blocked fallopian tubes. If fallopian tube damage is diagnosed at the time of a laparoscopy (Chapter 8), the extent of the damage should be determined, and the damage corrected at the time of that laparoscopy. If the damage is severe or if it cannot be corrected through the laparoscope, then IVF is the procedure of choice. It has been clearly shown that in the presence of severe tubal disease, IVF is more successful and more cost-effective than is major surgery for correction of tubal disease. *Don't have major surgery for purposes of correcting tubal damage--do IVF instead.* It's less invasive, less expensive and more successful.

While IVF was developed as a means of conceiving for individuals with nonfunctional fallopian tubes, it soon became apparent that couples with normal tubes could conceive with IVF. After all, fertilization can be achieved with far fewer sperm than were needed for any other approach, so it can be used to treat couples with male factor problems. (ICSI, see below, has improved the success of this approach even further.) IVF can, in fact, be used as one alternative for treating just about any fertility problem. Whether IVF or one of the other ART procedures is the best alternative is dependent on many considerations and is discussed in detail below.

GIFT (Gamete Intrafallopian Transfer)

Rather than a vaginal ultrasound approach for retrieval, a lapa-roscopy is required in order to do GIFT. The laparoscopy is necessary for visualization of the fallopian tubes so the eggs and sperm may be placed into them. Each follicle is again visualized, and the contents aspirated. After all of the follicles have been aspirated and the eggs isolated and evaluated, transfer of the gametes back into the fallopian tubes is performed. (The sperm sample from the husband is obtained prior to the procedure and has been fully prepared by this time.) Fifty thousand to one hundred thousand sperm along with an appropriate number of eggs (see below) are then placed into a small catheter, which is directed into one or both fallopian tubes. The gametes are deposited in the fallopian tubes where fertilization normally occurs. Fertilization does not take place outside the body in a GIFT procedure; the sperm and eggs are placed in the fallopian tubes and nature's way takes over. This entire procedure takes less than thirty minutes and is done on an outpatient basis.

While GIFT is typically performed via laparoscopy under general anesthesia, there are other alternatives. Good success has been achieved doing a vaginal retrieval and then doing a laparoscopy using micro-instruments under local anesthesia and transferring the gametes to the fallopian tubes, thus eliminating the need for general anesthesia. Also, some physicians transfer the gametes to the fallopian tubes through the uterus rather than through the fimbriated end of the fallopian tube.

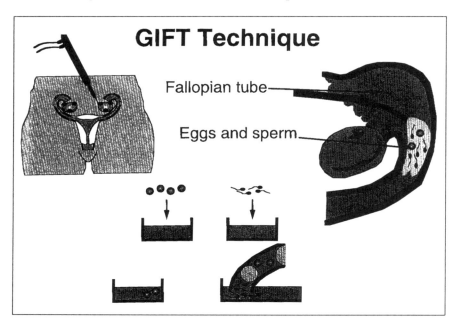

GIFT Technique

Fallopian tube

Eggs and sperm

GIFT differs from IVF in that we are placing the gametes directly into the fallopian tubes rather than bypassing the tubes altogether. The thinking here is that if the fallopian tubes are normal, and if we assume that the fallopian tubes can perform their normal functions better than we can mimic those functions in the laboratory, why not take advantage of this fact. Secondly, fertilization does not occur outside the body. In fact, the gametes are separated by a small air bubble and do not meet until they are placed into the fallopian tubes. This is very important to some individuals because of religious beliefs. Finally, the gametes are in the laboratory for a very brief period and embryo culturing is not required. As will be discussed below, GIFT does have a better success rate than does IVF, at least on a national average basis, and some of these considerations may account for this.

In order to do GIFT, at least one of the fallopian tubes must be normal. Any woman with at least one normal tube and infertility related to just about any other problem is theoretically a candidate for a GIFT procedure, although couples who have antisperm antibodies and those with severely decreased sperm counts are best treated by other approaches. There is one other aspect of doing GIFT that must be borne in mind: If pregnancy does not occur, we have no information as to whether or not fertilization occurred. If there is significant question about the fertilizing capacity of the sperm, either doing cryopreservation in addition to GIFT, or doing a different procedure, should be considered.

ZIFT (Zygote Intrafallopian Transfer)

ZIFT is kind of a combination of IVF and GIFT. Egg retrieval is performed via the ultrasound guided vaginal approach. The eggs are placed in the incubators, and a sperm sample obtained. The eggs are inseminated in the laboratory and are evaluated after fourteen to eighteen hours. If they have been fertilized, there will be evidence of this in the form of two pronuclei (the nucleus of the egg and the nucleus of the sperm)—this is a zygote.

Approximately twenty-four hours after the egg retrieval, a laparoscopy is performed (under general or local anesthesia) and an appropriate number of zygotes returned to the fallopian tubes.

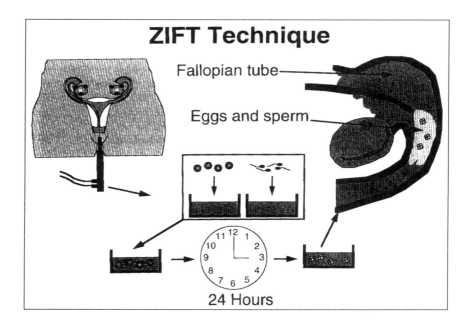

With a ZIFT procedure, fertilization is accomplished and documented in the laboratory, and the zygotes are then placed back into the fallopian tubes and nature takes over. ZIFT procedures are useful in cases of decreased sperm counts, in cases where there is question about the fertilizing capacity of the sperm and in cases of antisperm antibody production.

ICSI (Intracytoplasmic Sperm Injection)

ICSI is the most recent advance in ART procedures, having been developed only a few years ago. ICSI is a micromanipulation procedure in which a single sperm is injected into an egg. Prior to ICSI, there were many couples who did not have adequate enough sperm samples to achieve fertilization even under the most ideal laboratory conditions. ICSI has changed that! ICSI enables couples with only a few sperm (literally) to achieve successful pregnancies. If there are any sperm at all, ICSI is an option.

ICSI is done under a microscope using very carefully constructed microinstruments, known as *pipettes*. Using one instrument, a single sperm is picked up. A second pipette is used to immobilize the egg while the first one containing the sperm is used to penetrate the egg. The sperm is then injected directly into the egg. This procedure is repeated for each egg. Following sperm injection, culture continues and a zygote or embryo transfer is performed at the appropriate time.

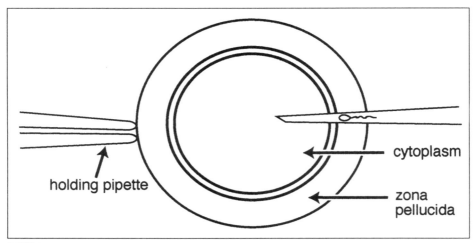

cytoplasm

holding pipette

zona pellucida

ICSI

CRYOPRESERVATION OF EGGS

In most cases, more eggs are retrieved than can reasonably be used for an ART procedure. If we retrieve ten eggs, and are only going to transfer three eggs (GIFT) or embryos (IVF), then some decision must be made as to the disposition of the other seven eggs. One option is certainly just to discard them since they are not fertilized. They are just eggs, and in an unfertilized state, they may be simply discarded. The other is to cryopreserve them.

Unfortunately, although techniques for the successful cryopreservation of eggs are being developed, the very poor success rates with this procedure do not yet allow it to be clinically useful. In order to do cryopreservation successfully, the egg must first be fertilized. Once fertilized, cryopreservation is possible at many stages of embryo development, ranging from the zygote all the way to the blastocyst. There are advantages to doing cryopreservation. The first and most obvious is that it provides an additional chance at pregnancy without going through all the medications and without going through another egg retrieval. Cryopreserved embryos are typically returned by a simple embryo transfer in a cycle using no medications, or at most minimal medications. In short, there's another chance of conception that's relatively easy and inexpensive.

There is another advantage to doing cryopreservation in the case of an IVF attempt—all the eggs can be inseminated. If one has opted not to do cryopreservation, then only a certain number of eggs can be inseminated because only a certain number of embryos can safely be transferred back to the uterus. For example, if cryopreservation is not an option and only three eggs are inseminated and only two fertilize and develop normally, then the chances of that procedure being successful may be compromised. On the other hand, if cryopreservation is an option, then all of the eggs can be inseminated, three of those that fertilize can be transferred to the uterus, and the remainder cryopreserved. Opting for cryopreservation increases the chances of the procedure being successful as well as offering an additional chance at pregnancy. Cryopreservation is also an option when doing a GIFT or ZIFT procedure.

SUCCESS RATES

A great deal has been written in both the medical and general press about success rates with the ART procedures. The information couples get concerning success rates is often confusing and, unfortunately, sometimes misleading. It is also somewhat difficult to compare success rates between the various procedures. There are many reasons for this confusion and difficulty:

Some centers don't offer certain procedures. For example, some centers may not do GIFT and ZIFT procedures, preferring instead to do only IVF. There are even programs that offer GIFT only.

Selection criteria differ from center to center. Female age is a tremendously important factor in determining success rates with these procedures. Centers that do not accept women over forty will obviously have a higher success rate than do centers that will attempt these procedures with someone over forty.

Some centers may have more success with a certain procedure than with others. If, for example, a center has the best success rates with GIFT, their IVF rate may appear lower because only the more difficult patients have IVF rather than GIFT.

National average success rates do not translate into success rates for a given center or even for a given physician. While national average success rates are higher for GIFT than for IVF, this does not mean that it is clearly a better procedure. A given center or physician may be able to achieve IVF success rates that exceed the national average for GIFT.

National average success rates for the ART procedures are determined from data submitted by all of the ART programs throughout the country to the IVF Registry. The IVF Registry data is very carefully defined, and the results reported to the Registry are subject to audit. This data is reported annually on a clinic by clinic basis and is an excellent source of information for any couple considering an ART procedure. The most recent year for which this data is available is 1995. The national average percentage of successful pregnancies per number of egg retrievals performed were:

IVF - 22.3%
GIFT - 26.8%
ZIFT - 27.7%
Cryotransfer - 13.3%

Any physician offering ART procedures should be able to provide a couple with detailed information concerning the success rates of their center. The numbers above are simply national averages. Success rates from center to center vary tremendously, with some centers now reporting IVF success rates of forty percent or higher, while others may have little if any success. The physician should also be willing to give the couple some indication as to how their individual circumstances will affect their chances of success. Age is one very important factor in this regard, but there are certainly others to be considered as well.

A couple should also check the experience and qualifications of the individual physician and the center offering the procedures:

- Is the center a member of the Society for Assisted Reproductive Technology, and do they furnish data to the IVF Registry?
- Is the center staffed by board certified reproductive endocrinologists?
- How long has the center been doing ART procedures?
- How many procedures has the center done?
- Does the center meet the minimal criteria for an ART program as established by the American Society for Reproductive Medicine?
- Does the center offer a full range of services including cryo-preservation, assisted hatching, and ICSI?

The decision whether or not to pursue one of the ART procedures is one that should only be reached after a couple has been provided with full information concerning the procedures. They should understand what treatments they must undergo, what monitoring and evaluation is involved, what procedures will be performed, what their costs will be, and what their chances of success are. In other words, be truly informed!

The decision as to which one of the ART procedures is best for a couple can be a difficult one. This decision must include consideration of the costs of the procedure, the invasiveness of the surgery involved, and the chances of success in the hands of your physician. Some consideration must also be given to how much, if any, of the procedure insurance will cover. It almost becomes a matter of balancing costs vs. benefits. If, for example, a particular center offers IVF for $5,000 with a twenty-five percent success rate and GIFT for $10,000 with a thirty percent success rate, then IVF may be the better choice at that particular center.

Another decision that couples must unfortunately face sometimes is whether or not to attempt a repeat procedure if the first one is unsuccessful. This decision can often be made much easier by discussing it with the physician. Following an ART procedure, the physician will have a great deal of information concerning the individual's response to the ovulation induction, egg development, sperm quality and fertilization, embryo quality, and perhaps even tubal quality. The physician can use this information to advise a couple if a repeat attempt is worthwhile. In general, unless there is some specific factor that would impel a physician to discourage a repeat attempt, there is good evidence that repeat attempts are worthwhile. Specific percentages must be obtained from your physician, but for virtually all of the ART procedures, there is data that the success rates justify repeating the procedure up to three times.

Finally, one of the most significant concerns over pursuing an ART procedure is the risk of multiple pregnancy. Everyone wants the procedure to work, and a singleton or twin pregnancy is wonderful. Triplet, and certainly quadruplet and quintuplet pregnancies, however, are not ideal. These higher-order multiple pregnancies certainly carry higher obstetrical risks, not to mention the demands they place on a couple after the children are born. This is a tricky issue. The more eggs returned in a GIFT procedure, the more zygotes returned in a ZIFT procedure, and the more embryos returned in an IVF procedure, the higher the chances that a conception will occur. But at the same time, the chances of a higher-order multiple pregnancy also increase significantly. These factors must be balanced when deciding the appropriate number to return. The age of the female is the most important factor in this consideration. It is not unusual to increase the number returned for women over the age of thirty-five, and especially over forty. The physician should be able to provide a couple with the data from their center concerning the number of eggs or embryos returned, the success rates, and the chances of multiple pregnancy. These numbers are tremendously program specific. Under age thirty-five, we very rarely transfer more than two or three eggs at the time of a GIFT procedure, two or three zygotes at the time of a ZIFT procedure, and two or three embryos at the time of an IVF transfer.

A SUMMARY AND PERSPECTIVE

To summarize, every couple must be comfortable with the procedure their physician has recommended, and this involves fully understanding how the procedure is done. Every couple must be comfortable with their chances of success, and this involves fully understanding the success rates of their center and their physician, and how the individual circumstances pertaining to any couple affect these success rates. And finally, a couple must be comfortable with the number of eggs or embryos that will be transferred, and this involves knowing how the number transferred affects their chances of success and their risk of multiple pregnancies. Get the information you need, talk it over with your physician and reach a decision as a team.

The ART procedures are tremendously successful procedures and have already helped tens of thousands of couples conceive. And success rates are improving rapidly. There are many programs now reporting successful pregnancy rates of forty or more per IVF procedure. With rates such as this for IVF, it becomes increasingly hard to justify more expensive and invasive procedures such as GIFT and ZIFT. And with success rates such as this, the treatment of impaired fertility has become more successful and more cost-effective than ever before. With forty percent of couples able to conceive as a result of a single IVF attempt, it is easy to see why IVF is assuming a much more preeminent role in fertility treatment. And it is easy to see why major surgical procedures, laparoscopies for mild endometriosis, and excessively prolonged treatment with, for example, clomiphene, have been relegated to the category of "the way it used to be done." The ART procedures have indeed revolutionized the contemporary treatment of impaired fertility, and with continued improvement in the success of these procedures, the revolution is not yet finished.

CHAPTER FOURTEEN
DONOR GAMETES

In spite of all the recent advances in treating impaired fertility, there are still couples in which one partner is absolutely sterile. The male may have no sperm. The female may be unable to produce any eggs or the eggs that she does produce may not be of good enough quality to allow much chance for successful conception. For these couples, donor gametes (either donor sperm or donor eggs) may be their only option for conception. For others, the alternatives available for potential success using their own gametes may be so expensive as to be prohibitive. For example, a couple with severe male factor may have to consider the cost of doing ICSI versus the alternative of using donor sperm. The use of donor gametes is a very accepted form of therapy. Over 30,000 couples a year conceive using donor sperm, and the use of donor eggs has become commonplace.

DONOR SPERM

There are no circumstances under which fresh sperm should be used for donor inseminations. The risk of infection (e.g., HIV) is just too real. All sperm used for this purpose should be frozen and quarantined. Donor sperm samples are available from sperm banks located throughout the country. Virtually all of these sperm banks are reputable, but there are some very specific guidelines that must be followed. We offer couples a selection of sperm samples from eight or nine different sperm banks. All of these centers adhere to the following guidelines:

All potential donors are carefully screened for any history of inheritable diseases and for a strong family history of health problems, such as heart disease. With any questionable history, individuals are excluded.

Any potential donor with a history of homosexuality, IV drug use, multiple sexual partners, or recent blood transfusion is excluded.

All donors are checked for HIV, syphilis, gonorrhea, herpes, chlamydia, hepatitis and strep. If this testing is negative, their samples are then frozen and quarantined for at least 180 days. The donor must then be retested, and only if all the infectious disease screening is again negative is the sample released for use. Frozen sperm obtained from centers that follow this screening and quarantining is safe.

The number of pregnancies that can result from the use of any one donor within a given geographical area is limited.

Certain nonidentifying information is provided by each of these centers. This information may include physical characteristics such as height, weight, hair color, eye color, and body build. Information such as education, occupation, religion, ethnicity, and even special aptitudes such as physical ability or special talents is also often provided. Some centers even provide photographs. We list all of the information from all of the centers in one notebook and ask each couple to select a donor who meets their criteria and characteristics.

Deciding to pursue pregnancy through the use of donor sperm can be very difficult. *A couple should never rush this decision.* They must first recover from the shock of learning that this may be their only alternative for achieving a pregnancy. They must evaluate the feelings that this generates in each of them, feelings that may include anger, depression, guilt and shame. They must evaluate their relationship, their parenting desires, their motivation in proceeding with donor inseminations, and their alternatives such as adoption or child-free living. Often, discussing these issues with a professional trained in this area is well worthwhile. In fact, we require that every couple who is considering the use of donor sperm or donor eggs meet and consult with such an individual before we will proceed. Each partner and each couple must be comfortable with the use of donor gametes before proceeding.

With proper consideration and evaluation before initiating donor inseminations, I have never met a couple who have regretted their decision. When they become pregnant, they are pregnant together, and they can deliver that child together. They have a child whom they can raise from birth (and take good care of during the pregnancy). They don't have to worry about the uncertainty of adoption.

DONOR INSEMINATIONS

When a couple is ready to proceed with inseminations, and has completed the required counseling, we actually have them select the donor. We do check blood types of both the husband and wife and ask that they choose a donor consistent with those blood types. Other than that, the choice is up to them. They simply look through the book and select the donor who meets their criteria. Samples from this donor are then ordered and kept frozen until needed by the couple.

Some evaluation of the female is indicated before proceeding with donor inseminations. Unless there is some previous documentation of normal fallopian tubes, I like to do a hysterosalpingogram (HSG, see Chapter 8). Donor inseminations are not inexpensive, and it is worthwhile knowing that the tubes are normal before doing inseminations. There may also be some beneficial effect in terms of enhancing conception rates as a result of doing the HSG. It is also worthwhile to be certain that regular and adequate ovulation is occurring through the use of BBTs and progesterone levels. This will allow the physician to decide how the timing of the inseminations will be determined. For women with regular, ovulatory cycles, the easiest means of timing the inseminations is with the use of an ovulation predictor kit (OPK). The OPK detects the presence of the hormone LH in the urine, which is present just before ovulation occurs. By simply testing her urine each morning, a woman can know when she is about to ovulate. When the OPK indicates, she calls the office and comes in that day for an insemination, and often the following day as well if possible.

Inseminations are done in the office. A speculum is placed in the vagina and the sperm sample, which has been placed in a small syringe, is injected into the uterine cavity through a small plastic catheter that is gently placed through the cervix. This is essentially painless. After lying in the office for ten to fifteen minutes, the woman can return to her normal activities.

Donor sperm samples are not inexpensive. Enough sperm to do two inseminations per month can cost anywhere from $400 to $700. The inseminations and sperm processing can add another $100 to $300 to this.

Anonymity. Donor inseminations are done on a completely anonymous basis. The donor has no access to the identity of the couple. The couple will have no access to the identity of the donor.

Confidentiality. Whether or not to divulge the information that donor sperm was used is a decision each couple must make for themselves. It is, however, incumbent upon the physician and the staff to preserve the right of the couple to make that decision. In other words, not even the obstetrician to whom they are referred need be informed of the use of donor sperm. Whether or not to tell the child, to tell their family, or to tell their friends is a decision that each couple must carefully consider. Again, counseling is helpful in this regard.

Chances. If the female has no fertility problems and is under age thirty-five, her chances of conceiving are excellent. Because the donor sperm has been frozen, the monthly chances of conception with donor sperm may be slightly less than with fresh sperm, but over a period of time, the chances become essentially the same. The chances are, of course, dependent on the woman's age, but in general are in the range of ten to fifteen percent a month. After four to six months of inseminations, about sixty to eighty percent of couples will have conceived. If conception has not occurred by this time, some investigation into other possible problems is warranted and other more aggressive approaches such as superovulation or an ART procedure may be indicated.

Risks. There are really no more risks associated with conception by donor insemination than by any other means. The risks of miscarriage, birth defects or any other type of pregnancy-related problem are not increased.

Finally, when you do become pregnant, consider ordering some additional samples of sperm from the same donor. Samples from a given donor are not always available. If you order additional samples from the same donor, you know that if you decide to conceive again, your children will be genetic siblings. These samples can then be maintained at your physician's office or lab for your later use.

DONOR EGGS

There are some women who are simply unable to produce any eggs. This may be a result of prior surgery with removal of the ovaries or prior cancer treatments such as radiation therapy or chemotherapy, which can render the ovaries nonfunctional. There are also a surprising number of women who undergo "premature ovarian failure." It must be remembered that all of the eggs a woman has she is born with—no new eggs are ever produced. It is believed that some women are born with fewer eggs than normal and that there are other women who use up their eggs more quickly than normal. There may be other factors involved also, but the point is that some women may reach menopause in their thirties or even in their twenties or earlier. When a woman reaches menopause, there are not any functional eggs left in the ovaries.

There are also a couple of other indications for the use of donor eggs. Women who carry a gene for certain disease processes, or who have abnormal chromosomes themselves may need donor eggs to allow a successful, normal conception. Finally, an ever-increasing number of women are delaying their attempts at conception until they are older. Successful conception until age forty and beyond is certainly possible. However, the older a woman is, the more difficult it typically becomes because of the effect of aging on the number and the quality of the eggs remaining in the ovaries. When efforts to conceive using their own oocytes fail for these women, the use of donor oocytes can restore their fertility potential to that of a much younger woman. There is excellent evidence that far and away the most important factor accounting for the age-related decrease in fertility is the decrease in the functional potential of the eggs. The uterus and the rest of the reproductive organs maintain their capacity to establish and carry a pregnancy until menopause and beyond.

At the current time, there are no "egg banks" like there are for sperm. This is because the technology that will allow the freezing and later use of eggs has not been developed. Eggs are very difficult cells to preserve through the freezing process, and the rate of success with this is so low that fresh eggs must be used in any attempt. Secondly, eggs are not nearly as easy to obtain as are sperm. An egg donor must undergo the relatively complex process of ovarian stimulation and egg retrieval. The use of donor eggs is, therefore, much more complex than is the use of donor sperm.

Potential egg donors are recruited by advertising or word of mouth. Any individual expressing an interest in being an egg donor must undergo the following screening and meet the following criteria:

1. We prefer donors between the ages of twenty-five and thirty, although donors up to age thirty-five are accepted if they have proven fertility. Although some programs allow college-aged women to be donors, we do not generally feel this is appropriate.

2. A very careful family and medical history is obtained. A strong family history of inheritable conditions such as heart disease, breast cancer or alcoholism, for example, exclude an individual. A history of significant medical problems in the donor herself will also eliminate her from consideration as donor.

3. Donors are screened for infectious processes such as HIV, syphilis, hepatitis, gonorrhea, chlamydia and herpes. Because donor eggs must be used "fresh," quarantining like that done for donor sperm is not possible. Potential donors are, therefore, carefully questioned about their sexual activity. If they have had more than one sexual partner in the last six months they are excluded. Similarly, if they have any history of intravenous drug use or other high risk behavior they are excluded. While this does not offer 100 percent protection against infection transmission, donors are by definition from a very low risk population and the risk of transmission of disease is extremely low.

4. All potential donors undergo careful psychological screening and evaluation, and standardized psychological profile testing. Their motivation is carefully evaluated. We have found that altruistic individuals make excellent egg donors while individuals whose primary interest is compensation are poor candidates.

The matching of donor and recipient can be done in many different ways. We have the recipient couple complete a "recipient profile." This details what characteristics and traits are most important to that couple. We also include a picture of the couple on this form, as well as their blood types. When a donor becomes available, she is "matched" to a couple by a panel of three individuals comprised of the nurse and physician in charge of the donor egg program, as well as the psychological counselor. The recipient couple is then provided with nonidentifying information about the donor and certainly has the right to reject any donor. Anonymity, however, is maintained. The donor is never identified to the recipients, and the donor relinquishes all rights to pursue the identity of the recipients.

Potential recipients must also undergo health and psychological screening. Particularly for older women, careful health screening including an EKG, chest X-ray, blood screening and general medical evaluation may be indicated. All couples requesting the use of donor eggs must undergo counseling and psychological evaluation of their preparedness for this procedure.

When a match is made, the cycles of the donor and recipient must be synchronized. The donor will undergo ovarian stimulation and subsequent oocyte retrieval just like that used for an IVF cycle (Chapter 13). If the recipient has no ovarian function, she must be placed on estrogen and progesterone in order to prepare the uterus. The use of estrogen and progesterone allows the physician to establish a cycle in which the uterus and its lining are in perfect synchrony with the cycle of the donor. If the recipient does have some ovarian function, she may have to use a GnRH agonist to suppress her ovaries before going on the hormone replacement protocol.

The eggs from the donor may then be used for GIFT, ZIFT or IVF (Chapter 13) depending on the particular circumstances and the particular ART program. Most programs have such a high rate of success doing IVF with donor eggs that other procedures are somewhat uncommon. Chances of success are obviously dependent on the procedure used and the ART program, but in general the use of donor eggs restores a woman's fertility to at least that of women the age of the donor. Whereas a woman aged forty-two may have less than a five percent chance of success using her own eggs to do IVF, her chances of success using donor eggs should approach fifty percent or more.

Some programs also allow women to recruit their own donors, or to use a friend or relative as an egg donor. This also works very well, provided that adequate counseling and evaluation of everyone involved are performed ahead of time.

Donor eggs are not inexpensive. The total cost of a donor egg attempt, which includes all medications, monitoring, laboratory work, egg retrieval and transfer and donor compensation ranges from $9,000 to as much as $20,000.

Obviously, appropriate consent forms must be obtained from both the donor and recipients. With appropriate screening, counseling and consent forms, this procedure is one that is rewarding not only for the recipient couple but also for the donor. Most donors have a real sense of satisfaction from having been able to offer another couple at least a chance to experience the joys of childbearing.

With proper consideration and evaluation before using donor eggs, I have never met a couple who have regretted their decision to conceive using donor eggs. When they become pregnant, they are pregnant together and they can deliver that child together. They have a child whom they can raise from birth (and take good care of during the pregnancy). Pregnancy with donor eggs also eliminates much of the uncertainty associated with adoption.

CHAPTER FIFTEEN
PREGNANCY LOSS

EARLY PREGNANCY MONITORING

hCG (human chorionic gonadotropin) is a hormone specifically produced by a pregnancy, and the detection and measurement of hCG form the basis of all pregnancy tests. hCG can be measured qualitatively (positive - present in amounts above a certain level, or negative) or quantitatively (the actual amount present measured) in both urine and blood. Blood tests are most commonly used for quantitative measurements because of their reliability. The presence of hCG can be detected within a day or two of the time of expected menses. hCG levels are used to monitor the early progression of pregnancies. *As a general rule, the hCG level will approximately double every forty-eight hours in normal early pregnancies.* If this rate of rise is not present, closer observation and testing may be warranted until the cause of the low levels of hCG is determined.

Vaginal ultrasound can demonstrate the presence of an intrauterine pregnancy as early as ten days after a missed period. This corresponds to an hCG level of approximately two to three thousand. Based on the initial hCG level, and taking into account the forty-eight-hour doubling time, we schedule the first ultrasound when the hCG level will be approximately five thousand. An ultrasound at this time answers several questions: Is the pregnancy in the uterus? Does it look normal? How many are there?

If the pregnancy is in the uterus, a gestational sac can be seen. This is a fluid-filled sac that on ultrasound looks like a dark hole. The gestational sac should contain a fetal pole, which is comprised of the early fetal tissue. Seeing a fetal pole tells us with a certain level of reliability that the pregnancy is probably normal. The presence of a fetal pole does not ensure 100% that the pregnancy is normal, but a relatively small percentage of pregnancies in which a fetal pole has been demonstrated will miscarry. Finally, we can see how many gestational sacs are in the uterus.

EARLY OBSTETRICAL ULTRASOUND SHOWING A FETAL POLE

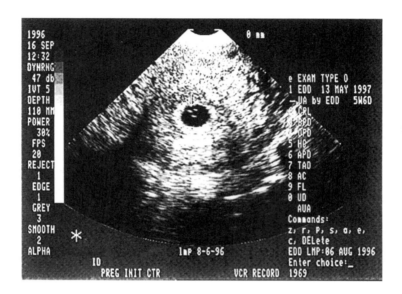

If the ultrasound fails to demonstrate a pregnancy within the uterus, an ectopic pregnancy must be suspected. If the hCG levels do not rise appropriately, the same is true. If the ultrasound demonstrates a gestational sac but no fetal pole, this is known as an empty sac, or blighted ovum. This is not a normal pregnancy (the vast majority of these have abnormal chromosomes) and is destined to miscarry.

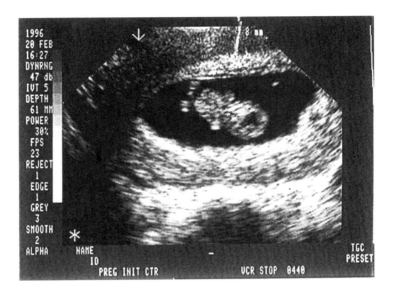

If an ultrasound performed two to three weeks after the first ultrasound, or four to five weeks after the missed period, demonstrates that the fetus has continued to develop and a heartbeat is present, the likelihood is very high that the pregnancy will be successful.

MISCARRIAGE

Miscarriage, or spontaneous abortion, occurs in about fifteen to twenty percent of all pregnancies, regardless of how they were conceived. Most early losses are a result of the conceptus being genetically abnormal. As few as one in three human conceptions is genetically normal, but most of the genetically abnormal conceptions are lost before the woman even knows she is pregnant. Even so, some genetically abnormal conceptions do survive long enough to result in a recognized pregnancy. These are often conceptions that have three sets of chromosomes (triploidy) rather than two, or conceptions that have an extra of just one chromosome (trisomy). These may present as an empty sac, or blighted ovum, which is a pregnancy in which there is no identifiable fetal tissue, or as a fetus that develops only briefly and then ceases. The human genetic message is very specific, and any variation from the normal set of forty-six chromosomes is rarely compatible with life.

Spontaneous abortion is, then, one possible outcome any time a conception occurs, and the chances are about one in five that any clinically recognized pregnancy will be aborted. And the chances do increase as the woman gets older. "Older" eggs don't divide as well when they get fertilized, and therefore the resulting pregnancies are more often abnormal. The chances of spontaneous abortion rises to as high as fifty percent in women in their early to mid-forties.

So how do we decide whether the loss of a pregnancy is just chance or the result of some other underlying problem that requires investigation? Most of the time, a single loss is attributed to "bad luck" unless some other factor is apparent. During their reproductive life-span, most women will experience at least one miscarriage. Should, however, two, or certainly three, losses occur without any successful pregnancies in between, evaluation is warranted. There are no hard and fast answers as to whether investigation should be initiated after two or three losses. The chances of another loss do increase slightly after two losses, particularly in older couples. Some investigation may be warranted at this time. After three losses, there is no question.

CAUSES OF RECURRENT PREGNANCY LOSS

The identifiable causes of recurrent pregnancy loss fall into one of seven categories:

Genetic

If the chromosomes of couples who have experienced three consecutive losses are analyzed, an abnormality in the chromosomes of either the man or the woman will be found in one to two percent of couples. There are many types of abnormalities, but the most common are translocations, in which a piece of one chromosome is hooked onto another chromosome (Robertsonian), or in which pieces of chromosomes are exchanged with one another (reciprocal). The implications of a chromosomal abnormality for the chances of a normal conception in the future are totally dependent on the type of abnormality discovered. If an abnormality is uncovered, counseling with a geneticist should be obtained to discuss its implications. Chromosome analyses are performed on blood samples taken from each partner.

Infection

While there is no question that infection can result in the loss of a pregnancy, whether or not it can cause recurrent losses is less clear. In couples who have experienced three losses, it is reasonable to treat both partners with a ten-day course of a tetracycline to eliminate infection as a possible cause. Cultures are not necessary.

Uterine Anomalies

Abnormalities in the shape of the uterus, which are also discussed in Chapter 10, must be excluded. When the uterus is abnormal, the chances of miscarriage are significantly increased. Much of this is probably due to the fact that there is not a good blood supply to the abnormal uterine tissue. If the placenta begins to grow on this tissue, it cannot get the blood supply it needs to survive. Uterine anomalies can be diagnosed by a hysterosalpingogram or hysteroscopy. Surgical correction of a uterine abnormality dramatically improves the chances of a successful pregnancy.

Another type of anatomic problem that can result in recurrent loss is an *incompetent cervix*. It is the responsibility of the cervix to stay shut and hold the pregnancy in the uterus until it is time to deliver. In some individuals, the cervix just does not form quite properly, and in others it malfunctions as a result of prior surgery or manipulation. An incompetent cervix usually presents with a relatively painless dilation of the cervix and premature delivery in the second trimester. An incompetent cervix can be diagnosed by history, X-ray and other simple procedures.

Endocrinologic Disorders

Certain disorders, such as thyroid disease or diabetes, may be associated with recurrent loss. Although other symptoms will usually be present to suggest these processes, it is worthwhile at least to check a thyroid-stimulating hormone (TSH) level to be sure the thyroid is normal.

Cycle Abnormalities

There is some evidence that individuals who have luteal phase insufficiency have an increased incidence of recurrent loss. This is certainly not to say that endometrial biopsies should be performed to evaluate this. Don't have repeated endometrial biopsies. But progesterone levels should be checked and the luteal phase evaluated. Progesterone suppositories or certain ovulation induction medications (Chapter 11) can be used to improve progesterone levels and the luteal phase.

Autoimmune Disorders

For reasons that are not clear, certain women can begin to produce antibodies to substances in their own bodies. One group of these antibodies are called antiphospholipid antibodies. The two most important of these antibodies are anticardiolipin and lupus anticoagulant. The presence of these antibodies is a well-recognized cause of pregnancy loss. These antibodies can be detected by blood tests. Treatment with low-dose aspirin (one baby aspirin a day) and heparin is the preferred treatment. At times, steroids may have to be added to the treatment, but the risk of side effects increases dramatically if steroids are used.

Alloimmune Disorders

In order for a pregnancy to survive, the female's immune system must recognize it as a foreign body, that is, one that is at least partially derived from someone else's genes. In pregnancy, this recognition results in the production of what are called "blocking antibodies." Blocking antibodies function to prevent the rejection of the pregnancy by the rest of the immune system. In some couples, the male's immune system may be similar enough to the female's immune system that her system does not really recognize the pregnancy as foreign, and therefore does not produce adequate blocking antibodies. Without blocking antibodies, the rest of the immune system can attack the pregnancy and cause it to fail. This problem is evaluated through blood testing which is rather expensive. Treatment involves injecting white blood cells from the husband into the wife so that her immune system will begin to recognize his cells as foreign and begin to respond appropriately.

Although some centers have reported excellent results with this form of therapy, *this is certainly the most controversial of any of the causes of recurrent pregnancy loss and should be discussed carefully with your physician.*

EVALUATING RECURRENT PREGNANCY LOSS

Recurrent pregnancy loss is one of the most difficult and emotionally draining problems any couple can face. Couples often wonder what they did to cause it or what they could have done to prevent it. While this is a very normal response, it has no foundation. *There are exceedingly rare circumstances in which a loss is due to something a couple did or did not do. Do not blame yourselves.* It may be bad luck or there may be some identifiable cause, but it's not your fault!

The toll that the loss of a pregnancy takes can be enormous, let alone repeated losses of pregnancies. It is perfectly normal to hurt after a loss, and the couples who do the best in the long run are those who go ahead and let it hurt, learn to deal with that hurt (this can take time), and then become stronger because of it. One of the biggest mistakes couples can make is to jump right back in to trying again before they completely deal with the hurt from the prior loss.

So when do we start to do some evaluation and initiate some treatment, and what treatment is reasonable? It is hard to justify doing much evaluation after only one loss unless the history of that loss suggests some particular cause. Beyond that, the answer is "it depends." In some couples, particularly older couples, at least some evaluation should be undertaken after two losses. Any couple who has three consecutive losses deserves some evaluation. They should be very cautious about conceiving until that evaluation is complete.

This evaluation should include:
1. Blood tests from both partners for chromosome analysis;
2. A hysterosalpingogram to evaluate the uterus;
3. Blood tests from the female for Prolactin, TSH, lupus anticoagulant and anticardiolipin antibodies; and
4. Evaluation of ovulatory function and the luteal phase, including progesterone levels.

This evaluation may include:
5. The sophisticated testing to check for the possibility of an alloimmune problem.

The treatment should include:
1. Genetic counseling for any chromosomal abnormality discovered;
2. Consideration of correction of any abnormality of the uterine cavity;
3. Correction of any other medical problems such as thyroid disease;
4. Initiation of low-dose aspirin and heparin if there is any evidence of an autoimmune problem; and
5. Ovulation induction or progesterone suppositories to correct any evidence of inadequate luteal phase function. Progesterone supplementation is often initiated even in the absence of any specific indication. It is safe, cheap, non-invasive and may be of some benefit until the placenta takes over producing the progesterone at about ten weeks into the pregnancy.

The treatment may include:
6. Treatment of both partners with tetracycline to eliminate any concerns over a possible infectious etiology;
7. Initiation of alloimmune treatment protocols, e.g., paternal lymphocyte injections. (This is very controversial. Be sure to discuss it carefully with your physician.); and
8. Cervical cerclage if there is evidence of an incompetent cervix. Cervical cerclage is a surgical procedure in which the cervix is "sewn shut," thus allowing it to hold the pregnancy in place. This can be performed as early as nine to ten weeks if the ultrasounds appear normal up until that time.

Once conception does occur, the pregnancy should be carefully monitored. An ultrasound done as early as possible will provide a lot of reassurance if it appears normal. In some couples frequent (even weekly) visits, ultrasounds and reassurance are well worthwhile.

ECTOPIC PREGNANCY

Fertilization occurs in the fallopian tube, and the very early embryo remains in the fallopian for two or three days before being propelled into the uterus by the fallopian tube. This occurs primarily as a result of the efforts of the microcilia, or small hairlike projections, on the surface of the cells that line the fallopian tube. If the early embryo is not propelled into the uterus, development can continue and implantation into the wall of the fallopian tube, rather than into the lining of the uterus, can occur. The reasons that embryos are not properly propelled into the uterus are not always clear, but are most often related to damage to the microcilia as a result of prior infection or insult.

The fallopian tube is by far the most common site of ectopic pregnancies, or pregnancies in sites other than the uterine cavity. Whereas the uterus is a distensible organ capable of expanding to hold a full-term pregnancy, the fallopian tube certainly is not. It is an organ that has very little capacity for enlargement. As the pregnancy begins to grow, its size quickly exceeds the capacity of the tube to enlarge and the tube will often rupture. This is the most significant consequence of a tubal pregnancy and can be a life-threatening event. Every effort must be made to diagnose and treat ectopics pregnancies as early as possible. (The methods by which an ectopic pregnancy can be suspected and diagnosed are discussed below.)

The two most commonly used forms of treatment for ectopic pregnancies are surgical removal and medical therapy with a drug called *methotrexate*. Surgical removal can be performed by laparoscopy in the majority of cases, and major surgery for this purpose is rarely required. Through the laparoscope, the surgeon can visualize the pregnancy within the tube and decide upon the best means of removal. If the ectopic has ruptured through the tube and significant bleeding has occurred, or if there has been severe damage to the tube, removal of the portion of the tube containing the ectopic may be necessary; otherwise, a more conservative procedure called a *salpingostomy* may be adequate. In this procedure, the surgeon makes a small incision in the fallopian tube over the site of the pregnancy and removes it, attempting to leave the tube intact. Recovery from either of these procedures is the same as for any other minor laparoscopic procedure.

If an ectopic is diagnosed early enough that the physician is not concerned about the possibility of imminent rupture, treatment with methotrexate is an option. The obvious advantage of this approach is that it avoids surgery. Methotrexate is a medication that has been extensively used as a chemotherapy agent, but pregnancy tissues are particularly sensitive to the effects of methotrexate. Therefore, very small doses of methotrexate with minimal, if any, side effects can be used and result in the cessation of growth by the pregnancy. The tissues of the ectopic pregnancy are then re-absorbed by the body.

When ectopics are treated conservatively, either by salpingostomy or methotrexate, care must be taken to be certain that the hCG levels continue to decline and return to zero. Pregnancy should be avoided for at least the next two or three months. The general incidence of ectopics is one to two percent of all pregnancies. The chances of an ectopic are obviously increased in someone who has had a prior tubal infection or prior tubal surgery. Following one prior ectopic, the chances of another ectopic increase to about ten percent, and after two ectopics the chances of another may be as high as thirty to thirty-five percent.

CHAPTER SIXTEEN
THE FUTURE

The good news is that the future looks brighter than ever before for couples with infertility. Developments in this field of medicine are occurring at a dizzying pace. This chapter will take a brief look at what the future holds and what couples can expect.

The ART procedures will continue to be the primary focus of research and development, with IVF leading the way. Success rates with IVF are high enough in some of the more successful programs that procedures such as GIFT and ZIFT, which require a laparoscopy, are already archaic. Pregnancy rates of over forty percent per IVF procedure, and over fifty percent per egg retrieval if cryopreservation is also performed, are possible now.

One of the primary changes in IVF will be the continued incubation of the embryos in the laboratory for a couple of extra days until they achieve the blastocyst stage of development (just prior to hatching). Allowing the embryos to develop to this more advanced stage will permit the laboratory personnel to make a more thorough assessment of the health and developmental potential of each embryo. This information will make it possible to transfer only one or two embryos to the uterus, thus minimizing the risk of triplet pregnancies while maintaining or even improving upon current success rates.

Micromanipulation techniques in the IVF laboratory will continue to have a large impact on this procedure. ICSI has already all but eliminated male infertility except for those rare individuals with complete absence of sperm. Preimplantation genetic techniques will continue to develop. These procedures allow the removal of a single cell from an embryo prior to transferring it to the uterus. This cell can then be analyzed for certain inherited genetic diseases and only those embryos that are proven healthy are subsequently transferred to the uterus. Gene therapy, introducing a healthy gene in place of a defective one, is also a possibility. Dolly the sheep has demonstrated to the world that cloning is now possible.

Monitoring and controlling these developments are the most crucial issues facing "fertility experts." These developments and procedures are occurring at a rate that far exceeds the ability to evaluate and develop guidelines and regulations concerning this new arena of human reproduction. It would be foolish of anyone to suggest that the possibility for abuse does not exist. Human cloning certainly shouldn't occur, but it is theoretically very possible. It is incumbent upon every individual dealing with this area of medicine to have a real "reverence for life" as posed by Albert Schweitzer, which commands that we be in full and deep awareness of the results of our actions, and that we take responsibility for those actions. We must police ourselves. Every couple should investigate, and be certain they are comfortable with, the ethics of any ART program they are considering when it comes to issues such as these.

The outstanding success rates associated with IVF will continue to change the whole way we approach couples with compromised fertility. We've already seen that major surgery for purposes of enhancing fertility is virtually archaic. Further developments in instrumentation will truly make infertility-related major surgery a thing of the past. We will be able to deal with virtually any type of pathology and do virtually any type of surgical procedure through the laparoscope. And there are really relatively few situations in which laparoscopic surgery is indicated at this time, and there will be even fewer in the future. As the cost of IVF decreases and the success rates increase, it will become harder and harder to justify doing even a laparoscopy.

New gonadotropins have been released at this time. Rather than being purified from urine, as all the gonadotropins in the past have been, these new gonadotropins are produced as the result of recombinant technology in the laboratory. (Bacteria are induced to produce very pure preparations of the gonadotropins.) They are of even greater purity and are administered subcutaneously. But there is some hope that we may not even need to use the gonadotropins someday. A lot of work is being directed toward just removing very immature eggs from the ovaries with a needle, and then maturing them in the laboratory, thus obviating the need for gonadotropin administration altogether.

Finally, there is the issue of insurance coverage for issues relating to fertility. A few states have mandated that insurance must cover fertility-related costs. But this is not the case in the vast majority of states, and in those states, couples are often left to cover all charges out of their own pocket. It is a shame that many couples find themselves unable to pursue attempts to conceive simply because they are unable to afford it—reproduction seems like it should be a more basic right than that. But the insurance companies contend that, first of all, infertility is not a disease, and that, secondly, the treatment of infertility is not cost-effective.

Whether or not infertility should be considered a disease is a topic for a book all unto itself: It may not be a life-threatening process, but it surely is one of the greatest stresses any couple will ever face.

In the past, there is no question that the treatment of infertility was very cost-ineffective. Multiple surgical procedures, prolonged treatment with "fertility" medications, poor ART success rates and the risk of higher-order multiple pregnancies all contributed to this. However, the treatment of infertility can already be cost-effective as outlined in this book, and it will continue to become more and more so with further developments as outlined above. We can only hope that by presenting this data to the payers that we can convince them of this fact and someday make it possible for everyone to avail themselves of these advances and this wonderful technology in their efforts to have a child and a family.

PART THREE:
MONITORING YOUR COURSE

As you progress through evaluation and treatment for impaired fertility, a great deal of information will be gathered. This section is designed to make it easier for you to record the results of your evaluation and treatment. You will find that keeping track of the information is invaluable. It will help you monitor your course and you will be better able to participate in your treatment decisions. If you ever change physicians, or seek a second opinion, having this information in one place will be immensely helpful.

We suggest you photocopy and enlarge the following forms for ease of use. Eight copies of the ovulation induction form and four copies of the ART form are suggested.

EVALUATION

MALE

Semen Analyses

Date _____ Volume _____cc Concentration _____ x 10^6

Total Count _____ x 10^6 Morphology_____% Nl.

Motility _____% Grade 3_____% Grade 2 _____% Grade 1_____%

TMNS_____

     Notes:_____

     _____

Date _____ Volume _____cc Concentration _____ x 10^6

Total Count _____ x 10^6 Morphology_____% Nl.

Motility _____% Grade 3_____% Grade 2 _____% Grade 1_____%

TMNS_____

     Notes:_____

     _____

Date _____ Volume _____cc Concentration _____ x 10^6

Total Count _____ x 10^6 Morphology_____% Nl.

Motility _____% Grade 3_____% Grade 2 _____% Grade 1_____%

TMNS_____

     Notes:_____

     _____

Post Coital Test

Date _____ Day of cycle _____ Medications _____

Hrs after intercourse _____ Motile sperm/hpf_____

Mucus:
Clarity _____ Ferning _____ Cellularity _____ Spinnbarkeit _____ cms

Notes:_____

_____

Date _____ Day of cycle _____ Medications _____

Hrs after intercourse _____ Motile sperm/hpf_____

Mucus:
Clarity _____ Ferning _____ Cellularity _____ Spinnbarkeit _____ cms

Notes:_____

_____

Date _____ Day of cycle _____ Medications _____

Hrs after intercourse _____ Motile sperm/hpf_____

Mucus:
Clarity _____ Ferning _____ Cellularity _____ Spinnbarkeit _____ cms

Notes:_____

_____

Sperm Antibody Studies

Date_____   Results_____

_____

Date_____   Results_____

_____

Sperm Penetration Assay

Date_____   Technique _____   Results_____

_____

Date_____   Technique _____   Results_____

_____

Sperm Function Tests

Date_____   Technique_____

Results_____

_____

Date_____   Technique_____

Results_____

_____

Date_____   Technique_____

Results_____

_____

Interventions and Treatments - Male

Date _____ Notes _____

_____

_____

Date _____ Notes _____

_____

_____

Date _____ Notes _____

_____

_____

Date _____ Notes _____

_____

_____

One-Month
Basal Body Temperature Record

Name _____ Date _____

INSTRUCTIONS:

1. Begin use of this chart on the first day of your menstrual flow. This is the start of your cycle, and should be indicated under the number 1 beside the word MENSES. Blacken this square, then additional squares, indicating your particular days of flow.

2. Above this blackened square, beside DATE OF THE MONTH, insert the date that your flow began.

3. Upon awakening each morning and before getting out of bed, place the thermometer under your tongue for at least two minutes. (Do not eat, drink or smoke prior to this as hot or cold substances will affect temperature.)

4. Accurately record your temperature by placing a dot on the proper line, within the square for that day.

5. Indicate days of coitus (intercourse) by placing a down-pointing arrow in the space provided.

6. Any obvious reasons for temperature variation (such as a cold, infection, insomnia, indigestion, etc.) should be noted on the chart near the temperature reading for that day.

7. Ovulation may be accompanied, in some women, by a twinge of pain in the lower abdomen. If you notice this, indicate the day it occurred on the chart.

MEDICATION INDEX

C   Clomid

HCG HCG Injection
PVS Progesterone
     Vaginal Suppository
P   Pergonal Injection

**BRING THIS CHART
WITH YOU
ON YOUR NEXT VISIT.**

DAYS of CYCLE ►	1	2	3	4	5	6	7	8	9	10	11	12	13	14	15	16	17	18	19	20	21	22	23	24	25	26	27	28	29	30	31	32	33	34	35	36	37	38	39	40	41	42
DATE of MONTH ►																																										
COITUS ►																																										
MENSES ►																																										
MEDICATION ►																																										
99.0°																																										
.8																																										
.6																																										
.4																																										
.2																																										
98.0°																																										
.8																																										
.6																																										
.4																																										
.2																																										
97.0°																																										

Note: Use a new chart for the start of your next cycle

Ovulation Kit _____ Estradiol _____

Ultrasound _____ Post Coital ____ _____ Progesterone/ HCG Check _____

Medications_____
Ultrasound Day _____ Results_____

DAYS of CYCLE ►	1	2	3	4	5	6	7	8	9	10	11	12	13	14	15	16	17	18	19	20	21	22	23	24	25	26	27	28	29	30	31	32	33	34	35	36	37	38	39	40	41
DATE of MONTH ►																																									
COITUS ►																																									
MENSES ►																																									
MEDICATION ►																																									

```
99.0°
 .8
 .6
 .4
 .2
98.0°
 .8
 .6
 .4
 .2
97.0°
```

Ovulation Predictor Change day _____   Progesterone Day _____ Result_____
Notes:_____

Medications_____
Ultrasound Day _____ Results_____

DAYS of CYCLE ►	1	2	3	4	5	6	7	8	9	10	11	12	13	14	15	16	17	18	19	20	21	22	23	24	25	26	27	28	29	30	31	32	33	34	35	36	37	38	39	40	41	4
DATE of MONTH ►																																										
COITUS ►																																										
MENSES ►																																										
MEDICATION ►																																										

```
99.0°
 .8
 .6
 .4
 .2
98.0°
 .8
 .6
 .4
 .2
97.0°
```

Ovulation Predictor Change day _____   Progesterone Day _____ Result_____
Notes:_____

Female Evaluation

Chlamydia titer_____ Date_____

Hysterosalpingogram: Date_____ Result_____

_____

Oil soluble contrast used?_____

Laparoscopy: Date_____ Findings and treatment _____

_____

_____

Date_____ Findings and treatment _____

_____

_____
_____

Prolactin level:_____ Date _____ Treatment_____

Repeat levels: _____ Date _____ Treatment_____

_____ Date _____ Treatment_____

TSH level: _____ Date _____ Treatment_____

Repeat levels: _____ Date _____ Treatment_____

_____ Date _____ Treatment_____

Other Thyroid evaluation: _____

Notes: _____

Day 3 FSH level: _____ Date _____

level: _____ Date _____

Clomiphene citrate challenge test: Date_____ Day 3 FSH:_____

Day 10 FSH: _____ Interpretation_____

Date_____ Day 3 FSH:_____

Day 10 FSH: _____ Interpretation_____

Notes and Other Information:_____

_____

Ovluation Induction Attempts

Date (day 1 of cycle) _____

Medication:_____ Dose_____

Day of cycle medication begun: _____

Ultrasound: Day of cycle_____ Results_____

          Day of cycle_____ Results_____

          Day of cycle_____ Results_____

          Day of cycle_____ Results_____

Estradiol: Day of cycle_____ Level_____

          Day of cycle_____ Level_____

          Day of cycle_____ Level_____

hCG given: Day of cycle_____ Dose_____

Endometrial thickness day of hCG: _____ mm

Progesterone level: Day of cycle _____ Level _____

Inseminations? _____ # _____ Semen values_____

_____

Date of pregnancy test_____ Result _____

Date menses began _____

Notes:_____

_____

ART PROCEDURES

Date:_____ Procedure:_____

ART Center:_____

GnRH agonist? _____ Dose _____ Started on day _____ of cycle

Gonadotropin dose:_____

Peak estradiol:_____ hCG given on cycle day: _____ dose _____

Endometrial thickness day of hCG: _____mm

Number of mature follicles on ultrasound: _____

Number of eggs retrieved: _____ Egg quality:_____

Semen analysis at time of procedure: Vol _____ cc Total count _____

Motility _____ Morphology _____ Notes_____

ICSI? _____

# of eggs transferred (GIFT): _____ # of eggs fertilized (IVF/ZIFT): _____

# of zygotes/embryos transferred: _____

# of embryos cryopreserved:_____

Progesterone level: _____ hCG level: _____ Date: _____

hCG level: _____ Date: _____

Notes:_____

_____

_____

NOTES AND QUESTIONS FOR YOUR PHYSICIAN

GLOSSARY

Abortion   The termination or loss of a pregnancy prior to twenty weeks of gestation. Abortions may be spontaneous (miscarriage), induced ("abortion"), or missed (loss of fetal viability without the passage of tissue).

Acrosome   Located on the head of the sperm, contains the enzymes necessary to allow a sperm to penetrate an egg.

Adhesion   Scar tissue, usually from one organ to a surrounding one; may form as a result of infection, prior surgery, or trauma.

Amenorrhea   Complete absence of menstrual periods.

Ampulla   The portion of the fallopian tube between the isthmus and the fimbria.

Androgens   Male sex hormones.

Anovulation   Complete absence of ovulation.

Antibodies   Protective substances produced by the body's immune system to help protect against foreign objects, e.g., viruses.

Antigen   Any substance capable of inducing the formation of antibodies.

Artificial insemination   Placement of a prepared sample of sperm into the female reproductive tract for to increase the odds of conception.

Assisted hatching   A micro-manipulation procedure in which a small defect is created in the zona pellucida to allow easier implantation.

Atresia   The process by which cells regress, die, and subsequently get resorbed by the body.

Azoospermia   The complete absence of sperm.

Basal Body Temperature Chart   (BBT) A means of evaluating the menstrual cycle by daily recording and charting temperatures.

Capacitation   How the sperm becomes ready to penetrate and fertilize an egg.

Cervix   The portion of the uterus that opens into the vagina.

Chlamydia   A sexually transmitted organism that can infect and damage the fallopian tubes. Few if any symptoms.

Chromotubation   The injection of fluid containing a colored dye at the time of laparoscopy to determine the patency of the fallopian tubes.

Clomiphene   An orally administered medication that is used to stimulate ovulation.

Corpus luteum   Once an egg is released, the follicle becomes a corpus luteum and begins to produce progesterone.

Cul-de-sac   The potential space located between the uterus and the rectum.

Cyst   A sac filled with fluid.

Day 1   The first day of *normal* menstrual flow.

Donor insemination   Insemination with the use of donor sperm.

Dysmenorrhea   Pain at the time of the menstrual periods.

Dyspareunia   Pain at the time of intercourse.

Ectopic pregnancy   A pregnancy located outside the uterine cavity, such as in the fallopian tube. These may be life threatening.

Ejaculate   The sperm, proteins, sugars, and other substances emitted at the time of ejaculation.

Embryo transfer   Transferring a fertilized oocyte through the cervix and into the uterine cavity.

Embryologist   A specialist in working in the laboratory with sperm, eggs, and embryos.

Endometriosis   The growth of cells that normally line the inside of the uterus in abnormal locations such as on the ovaries or surrounding structures.

Endometrium   The lining of the uterine cavity.

Estradiol   The principle estrogen produced by the cells surrounding the egg within the ovary.

Estrogens   Female sex hormones

Fallopian tube   The structure between the ovary and the uterus, responsible for egg pick-up, fertilization, and early embryo development.

Fecundity   The chances of conception in any given month.

Fibroid   A benign muscle growth within the uterus.

Fimbria   The finger-like projections on the end of the fallopian tube responsible for egg pick-up.

Follicle   The fluid-filled sac in which the egg develops.

Follicular phase   The part of the menstrual cycle from the time of the onset of menses until egg release (ovulation).

FSH   Follicle Stimulating Hormone - the pituitary hormone stimulating follicle growth and egg development in women and sperm production in men.

Gamete   The cells of reproduction, the egg in women, the sperm in men.

Gestational sac   The fluid surrounding a developing pregnancy - visible by ultrasound.

GIFT   Gamete Intrafallopian Transfer - the placement of unfertilized eggs and sperm into the fallopian tube.

GnRH   Gonadotropin Releasing Hormone - A hormone produced by the hypothalamus that controls the production of FSH and HL, thereby controlling reproductive function.

GnRH agonists   Medications that selectively affect the production of LH and FSH by the pituitary gland.

Gonadotropins   Pituitary hormones (FSH and LH) responsible for control of reproduction.

Habitual abortion   Recurrent pregnancy loss

hCG   Human Chorionic Gonadotropin - the hormone produced by developing pregnancy, very similar to LH and used to induce ovulation and stimulate progesterone production by the corpus uteum.

Hormone   A substance produced in one location that is then carried through the bloodstream to have an effect at a different location.

Hydrosalpinx A fallopian tube that is badly damaged and full of fluid.

Hyperstimulation Enlargement of the ovaries following the ovulation induction.

Hyperthyroidism Overactivity of the thyroid gland.

Hypothalamus The gland that controls pituitary function.

Hypothyroidism Underactivity of the thyroid gland.

Hysterosalpingogram An X-ray procedure allowing visualization of the cervix, uterus, and fallopian tubes.

Hysteroscopy A surgical procedure in which the inside of the uterus is visualized.

ICSI Intra-Cytoplasmic Sperm Injection - the direct placement of a single sperm into an egg.

Implantation Attachment of the embryo to the wall of the uterus.

Infertility The inability of a couple to achieve conception.

Isthmus The portion of the fallopian tube adjacent to the uterus.

IVF In Vitro Fertilization - the fertilization and subsequent early embryo development in the laboratory.

Laparoscopy A surgical procedure in which the abdominal contents are visualized, evaluated, and abnormalities corrected.

Leiomyoma Another term for a fibroid.

LH Luteinizing Hormone - The pituitary hormone responsible for inducing egg release and stimulation of the corpus luteum.

Luteal phase The phase of the ovarian cycle beginning at the time of ovulation and continuing until the next menstrual cycle. Progesterone is produced at this time.

Menarche The time of onset of menstrual periods.

Menopause The time of cessation of menstrual periods.

Micro-Manipulation	The process by which eggs and embryos are manipulated in the laboratory using instruments under a microscope (see ICSI and assisted hatching).
Obstetrician-Gynecologist	A specialist in the female reproductive system in both the pregnant and non-pregnant state.
Oligomenorrhea	Irregular menstrual cycles
Oligospermia	Decreased numbers of sperm
Ovary	The female gonad
Ovulation	The release of an egg from the ovary.
Ovulation induction	The use of medications and/or hormones to induce multiple eggs to develop.
PCOS	Polycystic Ovary Syndrome - a frequent cause of irregular or absent menstrual periods, it may be associated with increased production of male hormones.
Pelviscopy	Another term for operative laparoscopy.
Polyp	A growth on the internal surface of an organ, such as on the lining of the uterus.
Post-coital test (PCT)	A test to evaluate the interaction of the sperm and the cervical mucus.
Progesterone	The female hormone produced in the second half of the cycle, it prepares the uterus for implantation.
Prolactin	A pituitary hormone responsible for breast milk production.
Proliferative phase	The part of the uterine cycle corresponding to the follicular phase - during this part of the cycle the endometrium thickens.
Reproductive endocrinologist	An obstetrician-gynecologist with specialty training in infertility and endocrine disorders.
Salpingoscopy	A procedure in which a small tube is inserted into the fallopian tube allowing visualization of the inside of the tube.

Salpinigitis Inflammation of the fallopian tubes. Also known as PID (Pelvic Inflammatory Disease.)

Salpinigitis isthmica nodosa (SIN) Inflammation and destruction of the isthmic portion of the fallopian tube.

Secretory phase Part of the uterine cycle that corresponds to the luteal phase - during this part of the cycle the endometrium prepares for pregnancy.

Semen analysis The laboratory evaluation of a sperm sample.

Septum Tissue that separates an organ. In the uterus a septum is abnormal.

Speculum The instrument inserted in the vagina which allows the cervix to be seen.

Sperm The male gamete.

Testicle The male gonad.

Testosterone The principle male hormone.

TMNS Total Motile Normal Sperm - an evaluation of the number of sperm in the semen sample that are truly capable of fertilizing an egg.

Urologist A specialist in the urinary tract and male reproduction.

Uterus The female reproductive organ in which a pregnancy develops.

Varicocele A dilated vein around the testicle(s).

Vasectomy The interruption of the vas deferens, preventing sperm from reaching the ejaculate.

ZIFT Zygote Intra-Fallopian Transfer - the placement of fertilized eggs that have not yet begun cell division into the fallopian tube.

Zona pellucida The protective coating around the egg and early embryo.

Zygote A fertilized egg that has not yet begun cell division.

RESOURCES

The American Fertility Society
2131 Magnolia Avenue, Ste. 201
Birmingham, AL 35256

The American Society of Reproductive Medicine
1209 Montgomery Highway
Birmingham, AL 25216-2809
(205) 978-5000

Issue: The National Fertility Association
114 Lichfield Street
Walsall, West Midlands
WS1 1SZ
01922 722888
webmaster@issue.co.uk

NINE (National Infertility Network Exchange)
P.O. Box 204
East Meadow, NY 11554
(516)794-5772

Resolve, Inc.
1310 Broadway
Somerville, MA 02144-1779
617-623-0744
resolveinc@aol.com

INDEX

ABOUT THE AUTHORS

Dr. John C. Jarrett attended Princeton University and graduated with a degree in psychology. He completed medical school at Case Western Reserve University and did his residency in obstetrics/gynecology at the University of Michigan Medical Center in Ann Arbor. He moved to Indianapolis following completion of a fellowship in reproductive endocrinology at the University of Illinois. He has been Director of the ART Programs at Midwest Reproductive Medicine since 1985. He is board certified in Reproductive Endocrinology and belongs to the Society of reproductive endocrinologists, the Society of Reproductive Surgeons, the Society for Assisted Reproductive Technology and the Central Association of Obstetricians and Gynecologists. He has received numerous awards for both clinical expertise and teaching excellence. Dr. Jarrett has assisted in the conception of more than five thousand children and has performed more than three thousand ART procedures. John and his wife, Lisa, have six children. His hobbies include golf, gardening and fly-fishing.

Dr. Deidra Rausch started with Midwest Reproductive Medicine in 1985. She is a registered nurse clinician and spent many years as a fertility nurse. She obtained her Masters in Women's Health Nursing in 1988. Soon after, she became interested in teaching and the emotional aspects of fertility. Dr. Rausch has spent the last seven years counseling couples and individuals and helping them deal with the stresses associated with trying to get pregnant. Deidra recently completed her Ph.D. at Purdue University in Marriage and Family Therapy. She counsels both individuals and couples in issues such as infertility and self-esteem, infertility and the stress it can place on marriages, infertility and relationships with friends and family, and pregnancy loss. Deidra is nationally recognized as an expert in the field of fertility-related stress and its management. She is married, the mother of three, and her hobbies include piano, cross-stitch and golf.

OTHER INTERESTING TITLES FROM HEALTH PRESS

Popsicle Fish: Tales of Fathering
Michael J. Murphy, Ed.D.

Addiction: The High-Low Trap
Irving Cohen, M.D., M.P.H.

*Beautiful Again: Restoring Your
Image & Enhancing Body Changes*
Jan Willis

*In Sickness and In Health:
What Every Man Should Know
About the Woman He Loves*
Mary E. O'Brien, M.D.

Excitotoxins: The Taste that Kills
Russell Blaylock, M.D.

In Bad Taste: The MSG Syndrome
George R. Schwartz, M.D.